PSYCHOPHARMACOLOGY

A Concise Overview for Students and Clinicians, 2nd Edition

ARASH ANSARI MD
DAVID N. OSSER MD

ISBN: 1503171116
ISBN 13: 9781503171114
Library of Congress Control Number: 2014921067
CreateSpace Independent Publishing Platform
North Charleston, South Carolina

IMPORTANT NOTE: The information presented in this manuscript is meant to be an overview of some of the major topics in psychopharmacology and an introduction to the field, but not a handbook for the administration of available psychotropics. Specifics regarding clinical use of medications including doses are presented for educational purposes only. Although every effort has been made to present the material accurately, we cannot rule out typographical or other errors. As always, the package insert of each medication should be reviewed prior to prescription and administration, and treatment should be customized to the needs and characteristics of the individual patient after a thorough psychiatric evaluation.

PREFACE

Psychopharmacology, A Concise Overview for Students and Clinicians, 2ⁿᵈ Edition, is an updated and expanded edition of the authors' previous book *Psychopharmacology for Medical Students* published in 2009. Information about newly available medications has been included.

Although much of what was known about psychopharmacology and included in the first book is still current, this new text addresses areas of controversy and changes in emphasis that have developed over the past 5 years. The authors' goal in this edition has been to help practicing clinicians as well as students gain access to actionable information that may help them provide optimum patient care.

TABLE OF CONTENTS

LIST OF TABLES

INTRODUCTION

The use of psychotropic medicines to treat psychiatric illness has increased dramatically in recent times. Although the biological etiologies of most psychiatric disorders are still unclear, effective pharmacological treatments have been developed over the past 60 years that have become part of the standard of care.

Psychiatric medications are part of the armamentarium of most practicing physicians and prescribers, regardless of medical specialty. Although more severe types of mental illness are likely to be treated by psychiatrists, most prescriptions for psychotropics (e.g., anxiolytics and newer antidepressants) are written by non-psychiatrists (Stagnitti 2008). Psychiatric medications remain consistently prominent in the list of the top 200 most prescribed medications, and in the top 20 pharmaceuticals in terms of sales in the United States. From 2008 to 2012, medications for 'mental health' were ranked as the 3rd top therapeutic class (after antihypertensives and pain medications) in the number of dispensed prescriptions (IMS 2014).

As in the treatment of all medical disorders, a thorough evaluation must precede psychiatric diagnosis and subsequent psychopharmacological treatment. A complete history should be obtained and the patient should be examined. Medical or neurological etiologies that may contribute to the presentation of psychiatric illness should be identified and addressed. Nearly 10% of patients presenting with a psychiatric complaint will turn out to have a medical problem as the primary cause (Hall, Popkin, et al. 1978). Active substance abuse, if present, should be treated before or at the same time that pharmacological therapies are initiated. Obtaining collateral information from other treating clinicians and patients' significant others may also be needed in many cases.

Once a clear diagnosis is made, one should consider whether the condition requires medication treatment. Mild to moderate anxiety and depression often respond equally well to supportive interventions or psychotherapy (King, Sibbald, et al. 2000; Barkham and Hardy 2001; Cuijpers, van Straten, et al. 2009; APA 2010). Antidepressants may not be as effective as previously thought for the treatment of milder forms of depression (see chapter on antidepressants). On the other hand, if the psychiatric disorder or symptoms are severe, or if psychosis, mania, or dangerousness are present, then psychopharmacological treatments (and referral to a psychiatrist) are usually indicated. Although many primary care physicians may be quite comfortable with their ability to manage psychiatric illness, the amount of monitoring that is required to provide adequate follow-up should be taken into account before initiating treatment. When treating moderate to severe psychiatric illness, optimum therapy often includes the use of concomitant psychotherapy in addition to pharmacotherapeutic measures (Keller, McCullough, et al. 2000; Banerjee, Shamash, et al. 1996; Reynolds, Frank, et al. 1999; Katon, Von Korff, et al. 1999; Miklowitz 2008; APA 2010).

Placebo-controlled randomized controlled trials (RCTs), using strict exclusionary criteria when selecting subjects, have traditionally been used to study a psychiatric medication's *efficacy* (i.e., the ability of the medication to treat the condition better than placebo under controlled conditions). For example, studies comparing an antidepressant to placebo may use an 8-week double-blind parallel design and include subjects with major depression but without any other medical or psychiatric co-morbidities. Response may be defined as a 50% improvement in a chosen outcome rating scale. These efficacy studies also provide the response data that pharmaceutical companies must submit to the Food and Drug Administration (FDA) to obtain indications for developed drugs. However, in these studies, the use of exclusionary criteria and varying definitions of response limit their applicability to the general patient population, which often presents with more complex comorbid problems.

Effectiveness studies, on the other hand, are often larger, naturalistic studies that attempt to approximate 'real world' conditions by studying patients who may have psychiatric and medical co-morbidities, and by relying on broader outcome measures for assessing response. These studies may compare outcomes of treatment with multiple medications. As such, effectiveness studies complement our understanding of drug efficacy (Summerfelt and Meltzer 1998). Recent National Institute of Mental Health (NIMH) sponsored effectiveness studies have the added benefit of funding from a neutral (non-pharmaceutical industry) source, thereby avoiding possible study design shortcomings or evaluator biases that may influence study results (Heres, Davis, et al. 2006; Osser 2008). These studies include (1) the Clinical Antipsychotic Trials of Intervention Effectiveness (CATIE) (Keefe, Bilder, et al. 2007; Lieberman, Stroup, et al. 2005), (2) the Sequenced Treatment Alternatives to Relieve Depression Study (STAR*D) (Rush, Trivedi, et al. 2006; McGrath, Stewart, et al. 2006; Nierenberg, Fava, et al. 2006; Trivedi, Fava, et al. 2006; Fava,

Rush, et al. 2006), (3) the Systematic Treatment Enhancement Program for Bipolar Disorder (STEP-BD) (Sachs, Nierenberg, et al. 2007; Goldberg, Perlis, et al. 2007; Miklowitz, Otto, et al. 2007), (4) the Clinical Antipsychotic Trials of Intervention Effectiveness—Alzheimer's Disease (CATIE-AD) (Schneider, Tariot, et al. 2006; Sultzer, Davis, et al. 2008), and (5) the National Institute of Alcohol Abuse and Alcoholism (NIAAA) sponsored Combined Pharmacotherapies and Behavioral Interventions study (COMBINE) (Anton, O'Malley, et al. 2006; Anton, Oroszi, et al. 2008). Findings from these studies continue to influence clinical psychiatric practice.

Once the characteristics and efficacy and/or effectiveness of individual medications have been understood, students and clinicians can access available treatment algorithms and guidelines to help guide the choice of treatment for each disorder. Evidence-based algorithms, such as those of the Psychopharmacology Algorithm Project of the Harvard South Shore Program (of which one of this book's authors [D.O.] is the editor) (Ansari and Osser 2010; Osser and Dunlop 2010; Bajor, Ticlea et al. 2011; Tang and Osser 2012; Osser, Roudsari et al. 2013; Mohammad and Osser 2014) can be helpful in guiding and prioritizing treatments when multiple agents are available for the same condition. The latest versions of these algorithms may be accessed at www.psychopharm.mobi. Numerous international guidelines, for example those from the American Psychiatric Association (APA), the UK based National Institute for Health and Clinical Excellence (NICE), and the World Federation of Societies of Biological Psychiatry (WFSBP) also exist to help clinicians.

In clinical practice, multiple variables need to be considered prior to selecting a specific agent. The prescriber should take the following into account: (1) patient acuity and the need to address the most dangerous presenting symptoms (e.g. behavioral agitation, suicidality, catatonia, etc.) first, (2) the patient's past treatment history, (3) pre-existing medical conditions in order to minimize any increase in medical risk, (4) possible medication interactions, (5) the time required for amelioration of symptoms, (6) a medication's known side effects and how these may subsequently affect presenting symptoms, (7) the desirability of minimizing the use of unnecessary polytherapy, (8) possible pharmacogenetic factors and hereditary patterns of drug response and tolerance, and (9) financial cost-benefit considerations (Ansari, Osser, et al. 2009).

As in other areas of medical practice, the appropriate use of psychiatric medications is an art as well as a science. Art and science are combined when a clinician is able to support a patient in the acceptance of evidence-supported treatments with reasonable safety. However, sometimes the patient will have a strong preference for other that the ideal option and the clinician will need to be prepared to work with those preferences. The prescriber's relationship with his or her patient is of paramount importance. The patient's distress needs to be understood holistically within the person's overall life context. When the patient's distress is understood, subjective distress is often diminished, and therapeutic alliance and treatment adherence are more likely to be improved (Salzman, Glick et al. 2010). A "respectful posture that the physician is the student of the patient's life and illness" (Stahl 2000) can facilitate the treatment alliance.

Understanding a patient's psychology also allows the presenting symptoms to be better understood. Most importantly, a reductionistic approach to illness should be avoided:

"...chemistry (drugs) is not the solution for all human suffering. Not all unhappiness is depression; not all worry is anxiety. Not all restlessness is agitation, not all troubled sleep is insomnia. Not all feelings of unworthiness or low self-esteem automatically indicate the need for an antidepressant and not all exuberance and elation require a mood stabilizer. Not all difficulties with concentration or memory require a prescription of a stimulant" (Salzman, Glick et al. 2010).

Finally, given complex biological consequences (e.g., adverse side effects) and psychosocial implications (e.g., stigmatizing consequences of having a psychiatric illness and taking medication) of pharmacotherapy, the approach of the psychopharmacologist should be a cautious one.

In this book, characteristics of the major classes of psychotropics and their use in adults are discussed. Children and adolescents may tolerate or respond to these medications differently. The use of psychopharmacological therapies in these age groups is outside the scope of this book.

ANTIDEPRESSANTS

Antidepressants are medications that have been found to be effective for the treatment of depressive syndromes, including (acute and chronic) major depression and dysthymia. These syndromal states are characterized by the presence of depressed mood or loss of interest for most of the day (nearly every day for at least two weeks in the case of major depression) plus associated clinical symptoms (e.g., loss of energy, disturbed sleep and appetite, cognitive symptoms). Depressive syndromes are sometimes described as "clinical depression" to distinguish them from sadness that occurs in reaction to distressing life events. Antidepressants are not generally better than placebo or general supportive measures for treating depressed 'mood' alone when no other associated symptoms are present. However, lay misconceptions that antidepressants act as 'happy pills' are unfortunately still common.

Theories about the pathophysiology of depression are plentiful but none are proven. The inexact term 'chemical imbalance,' ubiquitously used or implied in the pharmaceutical industry marketing of antidepressant products, can be helpful in reducing the stigma of mental disorders by characterizing them as a biological (i.e., medical) illness. However, this term, which is best avoided in scientific

1

as well as doctor-patient discourse, is a gross misrepresentation of the complexities in the pathophysiological mechanism of depression. It also tends to obfuscate the psychosocial factors that may have contributed to the development of the depressive state. Antidepressants are only one aspect of the treatment of patients with depression and they should be used along with psychosocial treatment modalities when indicated (Cuijpers 2014).

Most available antidepressants primarily affect the norepinephrine and serotonin (monoamine) neurotransmitter systems (Nestler, Hyman, et al. 2009). Norepinephrine secreting neurons originate primarily from the locus ceruleus (and lateral tegmental areas) and project widely to almost all areas of the brain and spinal cord. Serotonergic neurons reside in the raphé nuclei in the brainstem and diffusely make contact with all areas of the brain. Antidepressants increase the available amount of norepinephrine and/or serotonin at the neuronal synapse by decreasing the reuptake of these neurotransmitters into the pre-synaptic cell. They do this by inhibiting the norepinephrine transporter and/or the serotonin transporter, or by delaying the metabolism of these neurotransmitters. Other antidepressants have direct effects on monoamine receptors. Genetic polymorphisms of the norepinephrine and serotonin reuptake transporters (Kim, Lim, et al. 2006; Porcelli, Fabbri et al. 2012) as well as polymorphisms of post-synaptic serotonin receptors (McMahon, Buervenich, et al. 2006) have been associated with differences in responses to different antidepressants. Once synaptic changes have taken place with treatment, long-term adaptations in post-synaptic neurons and resultant changes in gene expression may be responsible for alleviating depression (Nestler, Hyman, et al. 2009).

More recently others mechanisms of action have been proposed for the therapeutic effects of currently available antidepressants.

Antidepressants may increase BDNF (brain-derived neurotrophic factor) which may serve to undo the down-regulation of hippocampal neurogeneis that may occur secondary to stress (Masi and Brovedani 2011). Hippocampal neurogenesis, and/or the formation of new synapses, and re-organization of new neurons may also explain the therapeutic effects of antidepressants (Tang, Helmeste et al. 2012).

Tricyclic Antidepressants (TCAs)

Beginning with the introduction of imipramine in the late 1950's (Kuhn 1958), tricyclic antidepressants were among the first classes of antidepressants developed. They share a tricyclic structure (two benzene rings on either side of a seven-member ring), exhibit variable degrees of norepinephrine and serotonin reuptake inhibition, and are antagonists at several other neurotransmitter receptors (Yildiz 2002). Examples of commonly used TCAs include the tertiary amines **imipramine, amitriptyline, clomipramine**, and **doxepin**, and the secondary amines **desipramine** (metabolite of imipramine) and **nortriptyline** (metabolite of amitriptyline). All TCAs can cause the following adverse effects: (1) slowing of intra-cardiac conduction by inhibiting sodium channels as measured by QRS and QTc prolongation, (2) anticholinergic effects such as dry mouth, urinary retention, and constipation due to muscarinic acetylcholine receptor antagonism, (3) orthostatic hypotension due to peripheral alpha-1-adrenergic antagonism, and (4) sedation and possible weight gain due to histamine (H1) receptor antagonism. For these reasons TCAs need to be started at low doses and increased gradually, giving the patient time to accommodate to these effects. Individual differences in both severity of side effects and therapeutic effects (along with differences in therapeutic serum levels) (Perry,

Zeilmann, et al. 1994) do exist among individual TCAs. There is some evidence to suggest that TCAs may have strong efficacy in the treatment of psychotic depression (Hamoda and Osser 2008; Tang and Osser 2012).

The cardiac effects of TCAs have contributed to a reduction in their use over the past 20 years. Prolonged QT interval (called the QTc when corrected for heart rate) may be associated with torsades de pointes, a potentially fatal ventricular arrhythmia. QTc prolongation is also an issue with the use of many antipsychotic agents. All patients should have an ECG to rule out any existing conduction abnormalities prior to considering TCAs. Patients with recent myocardial infarctions should not initiate treatment with these antidepressants. In addition, TCAs (more so than other antidepressants) may be associated with an increase in cardiovascular disease even in those not known to have a cardiac history prior to treatment (Hamer, David Batty et al. 2011).

Most importantly, depressed patients who are at risk for suicide and overdose may not be appropriate for treatment with TCAs. It should be noted that a 1-2 week supply of these medications can be fatal in overdose due to the risk of cardiac arrhythmias. Therefore, depending on the patient's risk of suicide, clinicians may need to limit the number of tablets prescribed with each refill. This concern is significantly lessened with the use of newer antidepressants that are safer in overdose.

TCAs are often used for their mild to moderate analgesic effects in the treatment of chronic pain syndromes including migraine headaches (Magni 1991). These effects are independent of any effect on mood, with efficacy starting at lower doses, and with response seen earlier than when used for depression (Magni 1991; Max, Culnane, et al. 1987; Onghena and Van Houdenhove 1992). The TCAs, particularly amitriptyline and clomipramine, seem more effective for chronic pain than the selective serotonin reuptake inhibitor antidepressants (SSRIs, see below) (Ansari 2000; Fishbain 2000; Saarto and Wiffen 2007).

Monoamine Oxidase Inhibitors (MAOIs)

Monoamine oxidase is an enzyme that acts to metabolize monoamines, both intracellularly and extracellularly. Its inhibition increases the amount of the monoamines serotonin, norepinephrine and dopamine available for neurotransmission. MAOIs can act on two isomers of monoamine oxidase enzymes: MAO-A (found in the brain as well as intestines—it metabolizes all the above neurotransmitters) and MAO-B (found in the brain and platelets and primarily metabolizes dopamine). If an MAOI acts on both isomers it is termed 'nonselective'; it is 'selective' if only acting on one or the other isomer. Generally MAO-A inhibition is thought to be necessary for antidepressant effect (Thase 2012; Goldberg 2013).

The first MAOI, iproniazide, an anti-tuberculosis drug, was discovered in the 1950's. **Tranylcypromine**, **phenelzine**, **isocarboxazid**, and more recently **transdermal selegiline** (an anti-parkinsonian MAO-B selective agent that is nonselective at higher doses) are MAOIs active at MAO-A that are currently available in the United States for the treatment of depression. These antidepressants may be particularly effective for patients with depressive syndromes also meeting criteria for "atypical features" (i.e., two of the following four symptoms: hyperphagia, hypersomnia, a heavy leaden feeling in the limbs, and severe sensitivity to criticism or rejection) (Quitkin, Stewart, et al. 1993).

Although serotonergic side effects—see SSRIs below—and orthostatic hypotension can occur with MAOIs, there are two other primary areas of concern that limit the use of these agents (Lippman and Nash 1990). First, dangerous interactions can occur with certain foods containing tyramine, such as aged cheeses and red wines. MAOIs inhibit the metabolism of tyramine in the intestine, increasing its general circulation and ultimately leading to an increase in sympathetic outflow. This can produce an adrenergic ('hypertensive') crisis characterized by severe hypertension, headache, and increased risk of stroke and cerebral hemorrhage. Patients need to be advised regarding dietary restrictions before treatment. Also, to prevent a hypertensive crisis, MAOIs cannot be combined with medications that have sympathomimetic properties such as some over the counter decongestant cold remedies, amphetamines, and epinephrine (which is often added to local anesthetics as a vasoconstrictor).

Secondly, MAOIs if used concomitantly with serotonergic agents, such as SSRIs, may lead to 'serotonin syndrome,' a potentially fatal condition that is characterized by hyperreflexia, hyperthermia, and tachycardia, and may lead to delirium, seizures, coma and death (Sternbach 1991). The triad of (1) mental status changes, (2) alterations in neuromuscular tone, and (3) autonomic hyperactivity, (not all of which may occur simultaneously) must be recognized promptly and managed carefully with hospitalization and the use of serotonin antagonists (Iqbal, Basil, et al. 2012). To reduce the risk of developing serotonin syndrome, a two week washout period is required when switching from SSRIs (or any other agents with serotonergic effects) to MAOIs, or vice versa. An exception is when the SSRI fluoxetine is being discontinued: a five week washout period is needed before starting an MAOI because of the long half-life of its metabolite norfluoxetine (Boyer and Shannon 2005). Another exception is the new antidepressant vortioxetine (see below) which requires a 3 week washout period before starting an MAOI (PDR 2014). The prescribing clinician can and should access online drug interaction databases such as

DRUG-REAX® System (www.micromedex.com/products/dru-greax) or YouScript (http://youscript.com) to predict important risks of drug-drug interactions especially when considering the use of an MAOI. In addition to SSRIs, other serotonergic drugs that should not be combined with MAOIs include SNRIs (see below), TCAs, buspirone, triptans, cyclobenzaprine, dextromethorphan, and opiates with serotonergic activity such as meperidine, tramadol and methadone (Goldberg 2013).

Selective Serotonin Reuptake Inhibitors (SSRIs)

SSRIs are antidepressants with a more favorable side effect profile than TCAs and MAOIs and as such are among the first-line antidepressants. As their name implies, SSRIs inhibit the serotonin transporter from taking up serotonin at the neuronal synapse. Interestingly, polymorphisms at the promoter region of the serotonin transporter gene (SLC6A4) may influence response to SSRIs: the presence of the 'short' form of the serotonin transporter gene may be associated with poor response to SSRIs, whereas the presence of the 'long' allele may be associated with positive drug response (Malhotra, Murphy, et al. 2004) and better tolerability (Murphy, Hollander, et al. 2004). Data from the large National Institute of Mental Health Sequenced Treatment Alternatives to Relieve Depression (STAR*D) study, however, failed to support the association between this polymorphism and drug response (Kraft, Peters, et al. 2007; Lekman, Paddock, et al. 2008).

Currently available SSRIs include **fluoxetine, paroxetine, sertraline, fluvoxamine, citalopram** and its S-enantiomer **escitalopram**. Possible mild early side effects (that can be minimized by starting the SSRI at a low dose and increasing the dose gradually) include gastro-intestinal upset, sweating, headaches, jitteriness or sedation. Continuation of these agents may be associated with reversible sexual side effects (e.g., delayed ejaculation, decreased libido, or erectile dysfunction) in 2-73% of treated patients (depending on how questions regarding sexual side effects are asked) (Montejo, Llorca, et al. 2001).

Despite the relatively benign side effect profiles of the SSRIs as a class, they do have significant medical risks:

1. SSRIs have anticoagulant effects and are associated with a greater risk of bleeding syndromes especially if the treated patient is already taking non-steroidal anti-inflammatory drugs (NSAIDs) or corticosteroids. Gastrointestinal bleeding risk, for example, is increased 9-fold when an SSRI and NSAID are combined. This risk is markedly reduced with the use of protein pump inhibitors or H2 blockers (de Abajo and Garcia-Rodriguez 2008).

2. SSRIs are associated with worsening osteoporosis, increased risk of falls in the elderly and a two-fold risk of increased factures. There may also be some "confounding by indication" in that decreased bone density may be associated with untreated depression (Bolton, Metge et al. 2008; Ziere, Dieleman et al. 2008; Verdel, Souverein et al. 2010; Sterke, Ziere et al. 2012; Diem, Harrison et al. 2013). However, a recent prospective cohort study controlling for various confounders found no increased bone loss compared to untreated controls (Diem, Ruppert et al. 2013).

3. SSRIs may lead to hyponatremia, and may be more likely to do so than other antidepressants. The elderly and those already taking diuretics may be at higher risk (Movig, Leufkens et al. 2002).

4. Although SSRIs are generally weight neutral, paroxetine is associated with significant weight gain (Serretti and Mandelli 2010). Also, an observational study of patients

treated with SSRIs for obsessive-compulsive disorder found that both paroxetine and citalopram were associated with >14% of patients gaining more than 7% of their body weight versus <5% with sertraline (Maina, Albert et al. 2004).

5. Citalopram has been found to produce dose-related QTc prolongation. The maximum allowed dose has been lowered to 40 mg per day, 20 mg per day in the elderly. It should not be used in patients who are at risk for QT prolongation or who are taking other medications (e.g., some antipsychotics) that may also prolong QT. The effect seemed to be much less with escitalopram, the active enantiomer (Castro, Clements et al. 2013; FDA 2011). A recent large observational study did not detect any adverse effects from 60 mg of citalopram (Zivin, Pfeiffer et al. 2013), but another did confirm significant arrhythmia risk for citalopram—and escitalopram (Girardin, Gex-Fabry et al. 2013).

6. SSRIs may contribute to cataract formation (Etminan, Mikelberg et al. 2010).

SSRIs differ in their propensities to inhibit hepatic cytochrome P450 enzymes (e.g., CYP1A2, CYP2C9, CYP2C19, CYP2D6, CYP3A4) (Ereshefsky, Jhee, et al. 2005). Inhibition of hepatic enzymes may lead to decreased metabolism of substrate medications such as warfarin, metoprolol, tricyclic antidepressants, and antipsychotics. This may increase serum levels of these drugs and lead to increased risk of dangerous adverse effects such as bleeding, hypotension, cardiac arrhythmias, and parkinsonian effects, respectively. Among the SSRIs, citalopram and escitalopram, followed by sertraline, are the least likely to inhibit the metabolism of other drugs and are therefore preferred in patients concomitantly treated with multiple other medications. However, citalopram should not be used with other medications that can prolong the QT interval.

The relatively benign side effect profiles of SSRIs and their ease of use have contributed to widespread use by clinicians who might not have been comfortable with using earlier antidepressants such as TCAs and MAOIs. In cases of atypical presentations of depression, or depression in the context of recent substance abuse, SSRIs are more readily used even before there is absolute clarity in diagnosis. Under these circumstances, many clinicians believe that the benefits of treatment may outweigh the risks. However, evidence suggests that SSRIs are less effective, and possibly even ineffective, when compared to placebo in the treatment of depressed patients with concomitant alcohol abuse or dependence (Iovieno, Tedeschini et al. 2011; Atigari, Kelly et al. 2013).

Although empirical 'trials' of an SSRI (as an antidepressant with a *relatively* benign side effect profile), in situations where there is less than optimum diagnostic clarity, may be appropriate for some patients, the physician should still be aware of at least two other major areas of risk. First, all antidepressants can induce mania in the short-term, and overall mood instability in the long-term, in patients with a vulnerability to bipolar disorder. A clear family history should be obtained to investigate whether there is a genetic predisposition to bipolar disorder. Also, clinicians should be aware that younger depressed patients, who may go on later to exhibit manic symptoms, may be incorrectly diagnosed with unipolar depression when in fact they may have a bipolar diathesis. A pre-bipolar presentation of depression (Rihmer, Dome et al. 2013; O'Donovan, Garnham, et al. 2008) should be suspected in patients with (1) a family history of bipolar depression, (2) a younger age of onset, (3) a family history of completed suicide, (4) past poor response to antidepressants, (5) a history of treatment-emergent agitation, irritability, or suicidality, and (6) a history of post-partum psychosis (Chaudron and Pies 2003). Depressed patients with these characteristics may have bipolar rather than unipolar depression and therefore should not be reflexively started on an antidepressant (Ghaemi, Ko, et al. 2002; O'Donovan, Garnham, et al. 2008; Phelps 2008).

Secondly, antidepressants have been associated with an increased risk of treatment-emergent suicidality—this occurs in about 4% of treated patients versus 2% on placebo—especially in children, adolescents and young adults as noted in the current package inserts of all antidepressants. It is still unclear if this risk is significant in adults over age 25. The reasons for this increase in suicidality are not clear, although increased agitation (e.g., akathisia) or activation as a side effect (Harada, Sakamoto, et al. 2008), or the possible emergence of "mixed" manic symptoms (mania combined with dysphoric mood) in depressed bipolar patients as noted above, may be responsible. Despite the concern that antidepressants may infrequently increase suicide risk, it should be noted that overall rates of suicide in the United States had actually decreased over a prior 15 year span probably due to the increasingly widespread use of SSRI antidepressants (Grunebaum, Ellis, et al. 2004). Longitudinal data also suggest that antidepressant use is associated with a significant reduction in suicidal behavior (Leon, Solomon et al. 2011). Nevertheless, the concern about treatment-emergent suicidality argues for a need for careful evaluation and diagnosis, increased discussion of risks and benefits of treatment with patients (and family when appropriate), and close monitoring of all patients beginning antidepressant therapy. Prescribing antidepressants when indicated, coupled with these steps, is more appropriate than withholding antidepressants in unipolar depressed patients who are more likely to benefit rather than come to harm from these treatments (Bridge, Iyengar, et al. 2007). Unfortunately, surveys found that instead of the increase that was hoped for in the monitoring of patients undergoing antidepressant therapy (Morrato, Libby, et al. 2008), there was an overall decrease in the use of antidepressants and a recent increase in the overall rates of suicide (Gibbons, Brown, et al. 2007) after the 'black box' warnings about treatment-emergent suicidality were issued.

Serotonin-Norepinephrine Reuptake Inhibitors (SNRIs)

The SNRIs **venlafaxine, desvenlafaxine** (the major active metabolite of venlafaxine), and **duloxetine** are dual action serotonergic and noradrenergic antidepressants that would be expected to have efficacy similar to TCAs though without their anticholinergic, antihistaminic, hypotensive, or significant cardiac side effects. Milnacipran is an SNRI which is FDA labeled in the United States for the treatment of fibromyalgia but not for depression. Its enantiomer **levomilnacipran**, however, was released in 2013 and FDA approved for the treatment of depression.

Venlafaxine is primarily serotonergic at lower doses and has a dual action only at higher doses (Feighner 1999; Richelson 2003). Using venlafaxine at lower doses (i.e., less than 150 mg per day), therefore, should be presumed to be similar to using an SSRI. At higher doses it can have a mild to moderate dose-related hypertensive effect (Johnson, Whyte, et al. 2006; Mbaya, Alam, et al. 2007), although patients with effectively treated hypertension can tolerate venlafaxine without an increase in blood pressure (Feighner 1995). Desvenlafaxine is the major active metabolite of venlafaxine and has similar properties to the parent compound. However, the once daily starting dose for desvenlafaxine is equivalent to the target dose and no titration is needed. Also, its metabolism is independent of the cytochrome enzymes of the liver, and therefore no dose adjustments are needed in patients with hepatic illness (Reddy, Kane et al. 2010). These benefits over the parent compound, however, may not justify the increased cost of this branded medication for most patients. Duloxetine, which exerts a dual action effect throughout its dose range (i.e., not only at higher doses as with venlafaxine) (Stahl and Grady 2003), can also increase blood pressure, although the effect may be less pronounced and clinically insignificant (Raskin, Goldstein, et al. 2003; Wohlreich, Mallinckrodt, et al. 2007). SNRIs, like TCAs, are more likely to induce mania in bipolar patients than SSRIs (Leverich, Altshuler, et al. 2006).

Because low-dose TCAs have been shown to be modestly effective in the treatment of chronic pain syndromes, and SNRIs have a similar dual action, they have been proposed for the treatment of chronic pain symptoms as well. However, despite considerable advertising to the contrary, duloxetine does not have a clinically significant effect on pain symptoms in most depressed patients (Spielmans 2008). It *has* been found to be effective, and has FDA approval, for pain associated with diabetic neuropathy and fibromyalgia. Milnacipran, as noted above, has an indication for fibromyalgia but not for depression in the US. Although the more benign side effect profile of duloxetine may make it the preferred agent in a patient for whom the risks associated with a TCA are unacceptable, there is no evidence to suggest it would be more efficacious for the treatment of pain than the more cost-effective TCAs. Additionally, when used as an antidepressant, duloxetine has been found to be less tolerable overall than venlafaxine and the SSRIs, without providing any advantages in efficacy (Schueler, Koesters et al. 2011; Cipriani, Koesters et al. 2012).

Levomilnacipran, the newest available SNRI, is reported to have greater potency for norepinephrine reuptake inhibition relative to its inhibition of serotonin reuptake (Auclair, Martel et al. 2013). It also shows significantly greater selectivity for norepinephrine reuptake inhibition when compared to venlafaxine and duloxetine. It is not yet clear if these properties confer any clinical advantages over the other SNRIs.

Antidepressants with Other Mechanisms

Bupropion is an antidepressant with a poorly understood mechanism of action. It is believed to exert its effect through dopamine reuptake inhibition although it is unclear why this mechanism alone should provide it with an antidepressant effect. Some data suggest that it may also exhibit norepinephrine reuptake inhibition (Richelson 2003; Rosenbaum, Arana, et al. 2005). Bupropion has a different side effect profile than the antidepressants that significantly affect the serotonergic systems and can have mild stimulant-like properties. It can decrease appetite and is non-sedating. It is unlikely to cause sexual side effects or weight gain—two of the most common reasons for medication non-adherence in patients—and is reasonably safe in cardiac patients. However, bupropion can lower seizure threshold and is therefore contraindicated in patients who have a history of seizures or conditions that increase seizure risk such as eating disorders or active withdrawal from alcohol or benzodiazepines. The risk of seizure is dose dependent: this should be kept in mind when combining bupropion with CYP2D6 inhibitors such as paroxetine or fluoxetine that may increase bupropion serum levels. Among antidepressants, bupropion is least likely to cause mania in bipolar patients (Leverich, Altshuler, et al. 2006; Post, Altshuler, et al. 2006). Recent preliminary data suggest that bupropion, in contrast to TCAs and citalopram, may be associated with a *shortening* of the QT interval (Castro, Clements et al. 2013). Bupropion has comparable benefit to SSRIs for anxiety symptoms in depressed patients (Trivedi, Rush et al. 2001). It is a very reasonble first-line treatment for a wide range of depressed patients.

Mirtazapine increases both serotonin and norepinephrine at the neuronal synapse (and therefore like SNRIs has 'dual actions') through mechanisms distinct from reuptake inhibition. It is an antagonist at alpha-2-adrenergic autoreceptors thereby increasing norepinephrine and serotonin release, and it blocks post-synaptic 5HT-2A, 5HT-2C, and 5HT-3 serotonin receptors (Feighner 1999). (Mianserin, an earlier analog of mirtazapine marketed in Europe, has a similar mechanism of action). Mirtazapine can improve appetite (likely through 5HT3 and H1 antagonism) and sleep (through H1 antagonism). As expected, these immediate effects can be very beneficial in the treatment of the acutely depressed patient with poor oral intake and insomnia. Weight gain however can be a concern that might outweigh these advantages.

Nefazodone is a post-synaptic 5HT2 antagonist with weak serotonin and norepinephrine reuptake inhibition (DeVane, Grothe, et al. 2002). Although nefazodone can improve sleep, is neutral in regard to weight gain, and less likely than SSRIs to cause sexual side effects, it is used much less often since it was found to produce rare (1 in 250,000 to 300,000 patient-years), but severe, hepatotoxicity (Gelenberg 2002). This product was withdrawn by its original manufacturer but it is available as a generic.

Trazodone, an antidepressant structurally similar to nefazodone, is used primarily as a hypnotic (as it proved to be too sedating for most patients at doses necessary for antidepressant effect). Trazodone can commonly cause orthostasis and should be used cautiously in the elderly. Priapism is a rare side effect that should be discussed with male patients before treatment. Recently a new extended release formulation of trazodone with once-daily dosing has been introduced for the treatment of depression, although it is still unclear if this newer formulation would have any advantages over the generic compound. They both have no weight gain and minimal sexual side effects (Sheehan, Croft et al. 2009).

Vilazodone, a relatively new antidepressant, is both a selective serotonin reuptake inhibitor and a partial agonist at the 5HT1A receptor (Dawson and Watson 2009; Khan 2009). The 5HT1A receptor is a presynaptic receptor in raphe nuclei that is thought to be autoinhibited by increased serotonin in the synapse, so lowering this inhibition with partial agonism is meant to increase the serotonin reuptake inhibition effect. Also, 5HT1A is a post-synaptic receptor in limbic areas and in the neocortex, and partial agonism there is thought to possibly decrease sexual side effects. Therefore vilazodone is claimed to have a quicker antidepressant effect as well as less sexual side effects than SSRIs. However, it is not yet clear if either of these claims is true as comparative studies are non-existent. The side effect profile generally appears to be similar to SSRIs, with GI symptoms limiting rapid dose titration (de Paulis 2007; Rickels, Athanasiou et al. 2009; Khan, Cutler et al. 2011; Laughren, Gobburu et al. 2011). There is insufficient evidence to recommend this newer drug over less expensive alternatives.

Vortioxetine was FDA-approved in 2013. It is referred to as a 'multimodal' antidepressant with a wide range of neurotransmitter and receptor effects (Mork, Montezinho et al. 2013). In addition to inhibiting the serotonin transporter, it is an antagonist at 5HT1D,

5HT3, 5HT7 receptors, a partial agonist at the 5HT1B receptor, and a full agonist at the 5HT1A receptor. Based on animal studies, it is postulated to have a positive effect on memory and attention due to its antagonism at the 5HT7 receptor but this effect has not yet been established in humans. Results of controlled trials for efficacy in depression are mixed (Jain, Mahableshwarkar et al. 2013; Citrome 2014). Nausea may be a common adverse effect. As with vilazodone there is insufficient evidence at this time to recommend its use over already available and less costly antidepressants.

Starting, Continuing, and Terminating Antidepressant Treatment

Once the decision has been made to start an antidepressant, the starting dose should be a low dose to minimize adverse effects. It is then titrated as tolerated to a therapeutic dose. Response may begin by the end of the first week, but generally 2-6 weeks of treatment are needed for a more substantial response (Taylor, Freemantle et al. 2006). Full response in the first week is possible, but it could be a placebo response or the sign of a possible manic switch, the latter suggesting the advisability of discontinuing the antidepressant. Other typical side effects of antidepressants can occur in the first days of treatment; some may even target and alleviate certain depression symptoms. For example, the sleep and appetite enhancing effects of mirtazapine, which can be seen early in treatment, are likely to be helpful to a patient who has been suffering from insomnia and poor oral intake because of his or her depression. Such an antidepressant then could help a patient *symptomatically* feel better within the first few days. However, the onset of effects on the core symptoms of depression may still require several weeks. If no improvement, no matter how small, is seen by 2-4 weeks (or 1-2 weeks in the inpatient setting), then an increase in dose (if appropriate), or a change of antidepressant, is likely to be warranted. Once improvement begins however, gradual subtle changes in mood, affect, and cognition may then continue for the duration of the medication trial which may take up to 12 weeks.

Patients who respond to treatment and have had only one depressive episode are often recommended to remain on the antidepressant for 9-12 months before considering discontinuation. However, if there have been repeated depressive episodes or a history of suicidality or other dangerousness, a longer period of many years of continuation treatment is usually recommended. Although questions have been raised about the effectiveness of antidepressants in treating acute depression (see below discussion), there is less question about the benefits of antidepressants in relapse prevention (Geddes, Carney et al. 2003; Glue, Donovan et al. 2010).

If a decision is made to discontinue antidepressant treatment, the medication should be tapered off slowly, particularly to avoid the occurrence of an 'SSRI discontinuation syndrome.' This is particularly true when tapering off paroxetine or venlafaxine. The discontinuation syndrome is characterized by vague neurological symptoms, dizziness, GI symptoms, headache and flu-like symptoms. It is generally mild, lasting a few days to a few weeks and can be reversed by re-introducing the withdrawn agent (Haddad 1998). The syndrome is not known generally to be life threatening, but in some individuals it can be extremely distressing. Often patients assume that the symptoms indicate that their depression is returning: they should be reassured that these immediate symptoms are probably withdrawal-related and they may wait to see if an actual mood syndrome re-develops over the coming months.

Do Antidepressants Work?

Although numerous published randomized controlled trials comparing individual antidepressants with placebo have historically shown antidepressants to be superior to placebo (50-60s% over 30-40s%), concerns have been raised about the overall clinical effectiveness of these medications. First, there is the concern that data are selectively published, so that many studies unfavorable to the studied antidepressants may have never been publicly reported, thus biasing the evidence-base. A review of antidepressant effect size including data from published *and* unpublished studies (available to the FDA) showed a lower antidepressant effect size than that derived from reviews of published literature only (Turner, Matthews et al. 2008). This lower effect size has been described as "clinically insignificant" (Kirsch, Deacon et al. 2008; Turner and Rosenthal 2008). One of the reasons for the marginal net efficacy is an increasing placebo response rate in the more recent antidepressant efficacy studies (Walsh, Seidman et al. 2002). These rates may be a result of the recruitment of more mildly ill subjects in clinical trials, leading to a greater likelihood of a placebo response in less ill patients. Some analyses have found that patients who are only mildly to moderately ill do not respond better to antidepressants than to placebo, but as severity increases the benefits become significant (Kirsch, Deacon et al. 2008; Khin, Chen et al. 2011). However, a more recent review of data on fluoxetine and venlafaxine found benefit at all levels of severity (Gibbons, Hur et al. 2012). In summary, antidepressants may still be efficacious, but perhaps not as often as previously thought, and they may be more likely to be clinically effective in the severely depressed. However, some would assert that problems with research conduct and design, rather than problems with the medications, account for most of the disappointing outcomes.

Further Notes on the Clinical Use of Antidepressants

First-line Treatments: Clinical practice today emphasizes the use of newer ('second generation') antidepressants including SSRIs, SNRIs, bupropion, and mirtazapine. As discussed above, the older tricyclics and MAOIs are not first-line because of their greater toxicity and risk of harm from overdose. In a meta-analysis of 203 studies comparing the efficacy and side effects of these newer antidepressants, no substantial differences in effectiveness were found (Gartlehner, Gaynes, et al. 2008). The authors recommended that antidepressants be selected on the basis of differences in expected side effects and cost (i.e. – use generic products over brand items). Another review of 117 trials concluded that sertraline had the most favorable balance among benefits, side effects, and acquisition cost (Cipriani, Furukawa, et al. 2009). Escitalopram also had slightly better efficacy, but was still an expensive brand product at the time of the study. It has subsequently become available in generic form, and the cost has become much lower in some practice settings. Paroxetine and mirtazapine are often avoided as first-line choices if weight gain is an important consideration, as it often is.

Outcome Studies: The STAR*D study (Sequenced Treatment Alternatives to Relieve Depression), sponsored by the NIMH was a study of medications for the treatment of major depression. It produced important insights into the optimum use of pharmacotherapy for this disorder (Wisniewski, Rush et al. 2009). STAR*D started with almost 4,000 heterogeneous "real world" patients with major depression, who were treated by a mixture of psychiatrists and primary care physicians. Patients agreed to have up to 4 sequential medication trials with the goal of achieving remission from their depression. Each trial lasted up to 14 weeks. Patients started with citalopram for the first trial. If response was unsatisfactory, they could have a switch to one of three antidepressants, or an augmentation with one of two augmenting agents. For the third trial, there were other switches or augmentations available, and finally for those still depressed and still willing to undergo the fourth trial, there was the choice of an MAOI or a combination of venlafaxine and mirtazapine. The latter combination has been referred to informally as 'rocket fuel' because of the four different neurotransmitter alterations that it is thought to induce (McGrath, Stewart, et al. 2006). Key findings from STAR*D include the following:

- Citalopram did not work well if patients met the DSM-IV criteria for melancholic features (McGrath, Khan, et al. 2008).
- The switches in the second trial (to another SSRI: sertraline, to bupropion, or to venlafaxine) had equal efficacy.
- The augmentations in the second trial (buspirone--discussed in the anxiolytic section below--or bupropion) worked equally well.
- *Nothing* worked well in trials one or two if patients had significant anxiety symptoms along with their depression (Fava, Rush, et al. 2008). However, a recent study with adjunctive aripiprazole (an antipsychotic discussed below) added to an SSRI found good results in patients with depression mixed with anxiety, in a post-hoc analysis (Trivedi, Thase, et al. 2008). This needs replication in a prospectively designed study with comparison to other augmentations.
- In the third trial, switching to a TCA worked fairly well. It might have worked better if clinicians had dosed the TCA properly and used plasma levels to monitor adequacy of dosage.

- Adding lithium (discussed in the mood stabilizer section below) did not work as well as adding triiodothyronine (T3) in the third trial, but lithium might have done better if clinicians had dosed it properly.

- In trial 4, the MAOI did not do well compared to the venlafaxine/mirtazapine combination, but clinicians underdosed the MAOI. Unfortunately, for the few patients who improved from either treatment, early relapse was common.

As a group, STAR*D subjects were not particularly interested in psychotherapeutic treatment for their depression. Psychotherapy was available as an option in the second treatment trial, but patients could elect to drop it from the option list and most did so (Wisniewski, Fava, et al. 2007). The modest remission rates seen in STAR*D may reflect that a major component of the improvement in depression seen in research and clinical settings comes from the non-specific, interpersonal supportive aspects of care including the therapeutic alliance. STAR*D patients might have been less susceptible to these benefits than other patients who are more invested in psychosocial treatments of their disorder. It is hoped that future studies will improve our ability to select the best treatments for each patient, psychopharmacological and psychotherapeutic, depending on their needs and preferences.

Monotherapy vs. Combination Antidepressants

There has been much recent interest in the possibility that a combination of two or more antidepressants might benefit a wider spectrum of patients or work more rapidly than a single agent like an SSRI or bupropion (Blier, Ward et al. 2010). However, the

Combining Medications to Enhance Depression Outcomes (CO-MED) study seemed to settle the issue in favor of monotherapy (Rush, Trivedi et al. 2011; Sung, Haley et al. 2012). Six hundred sixty-five outpatients were treated in psychiatric and primary care sites. They were randomized to either escitalopram 10-20 mg daily, escitalopram plus bupropion, or mirtazapine plus venlafaxine. At 12 weeks, remission rates were 39% for the first two options and 38% for the 'rocket fuel' combination, which had worse adverse effects. The study implied that escitalopram may be a particularly good monotherapy to select initially. However given its sexual side effects, many patients may still prefer to start with bupropion monotherapy (not an option in CO-MED).

Future Trends

The latest available antidepressants have been 'me too' drugs, seeming to offer same results through fairly similar mechanisms of action. However, some recent research has increased interest in novel agents for the treatment of depression:

1. Ketamine, a rapid-acting N-methyl-D-aspartate glutamate receptor antagonist, may have antidepressant effects. The proposed mechanism of action is through an increase in synaptogenesis in the medial prefrontal cortex. Although much of the evidence for ketamine is in the treatment of bipolar depression (see chapter on mood stabilizers), there is some evidence to suggest a role in the treatment of unipolar depression as well, and particularly in treatment resistant depression. Most notably, it has been observed that ketamine can produce a rapid response within 2 hours after a single intravenous infusion, and the effect can last up to a week (Zarate, Singh et al. 2006; Covvey, Crawford et al. 2012; Mathew, Shah et al. 2012). It is not

yet clear if the response can be sustained over the longer term. Preliminary evidence also suggests a possible role for ketamine in decreasing suicidal ideation (Larkin and Beautrais 2011). Studies with inhaled preparations of ketamine have been reported at meetings and may be a more practical method for sustained administration.

2. Agomelatine and ramelteon are MT1 and MT2 melatonin receptor agonists. Agomelatine is also a 5HT2C receptor antagonist and may increase noradrenaline and dopamine release in the frontal cortex. Although the evidence is mixed, there is some evidence that agomelatine can help alleviate depression in addition to improving disturbed sleep (Kasper 2009; Hickie and Rogers 2011). However, it so far has not been approved for use in the United States.

Table of Antidepressants

Table 1 summarizes characteristics of commonly used antidepressants (Ansari and Osser 2009; WHO 2011; PDR 2014).

TABLE 1. COMMONLY USED ANTIDEPRESSANTS

MEDICATION*	DOSING**	COMMENTS/ *FDA Indication*
Imipramine (TCA) (Tofranil®)	See nortriptyline, except increase gradually to 100-200 mg po qhs	Check baseline ECG; therapeutic serum level of imipramine + its metabolite desipramine: 175-350 ng/mL; TCA most commonly used in comparative anxiety studies; CYP1A2. CYP2D6 substrate. *Depression/Temporary adjunct in childhood enuresis in patients greater or equal to 6 years of age*
Amitriptyline (TCA) (Elavil®)	See nortriptyline, except increase gradually to 100-200 mg po qhs	Check baseline ECG; possible therapeutic serum level of amitriptyline + its metabolite nortriptyline: 93-140 ng/mL; frequently used in low doses for chronic pain; most anticholinergic TCA; TCA with most overall adverse effects; CYP1A2, CYP2D6 substrate. On WHO Essential Medicines List for depressive disorders. *Depression*
Clomipramine (TCA) (Anafranil®)	See nortriptyline, except increase gradually to 100-200 mg po qhs	Check baseline ECG; most serotonergic TCA; CYP1A2, CYP2D6 substrate. Effective in low doses for chronic pain. On WHO Essential Medicines List for OCD. *OCD*
Doxepin (TCA) (Sinequan®, Adapin®, Silenor®)	See nortriptyline, except increase gradually to 100-200 mg po qhs	Check baseline ECG; very sedating TCA, usually used as adjunct for insomnia;

	Newly marketed as a hypnotic in doses of 3 and 6 mg nightly (Silenor®)	CYP2D6 substrate. *Depression/Anxiety* For Silenor®: *Insomnia characterized by difficulties with sleep maintenance*
Desipramine (TCA) (Norpramin®)	See nortriptyline, except give in am and/or in divided doses, gradually increase to 100-200 mg/day	Check baseline ECG; serum therapeutic level of desipramine: greater than 115 ng/mL; least sedating (possibly activating) TCA; most noradrenergic TCA; CYP2D6 substrate. *Depression*
Nortriptyline (TCA) (Aventyl®, Pamelor®)	Start: 10-25 mg po qhs and increase by 10-25 mg every 2 days until 50-150 mg/day in divided doses then check serum level	Check baseline ECG; therapeutic serum level of nortriptyline: 58-148 ng/mL (TCA with most defined serum level—inverted U dose-response curve); TCA with least postural hypotension so best for use in elderly; CYP2D6 substrate. *Depression*
Phenelzine (MAOI) (Nardil®)	Start: 15 mg po bid and increase weekly by 15 mg/day to 45-60 mg/ day	Nonselective MAOI; dangerous medication and food interactions (see package insert). *Atypical and other depressions not responsive to other antidepressants*
Tranylcypromine (MAOI) (Parnate®)	Start: 10 mg po bid and increase weekly by 10 mg/day to 30-60 mg/day	Nonselective MAOI; dangerous food and drug interactions (see package insert). *MDD without melancholia*
Transdermal	Start: 6 mg transdermal q	Selective MAO-B inhibitor;

Selegiline (MAOI) (Emsam®)	day then increase by 3 mg patches as needed to max of 12 mg/day	at 6 mg dose may not need diet restrictions (but perhaps with less antidepressant effect), but at higher doses a nonselective MAOI and needs diet restrictions; dangerous food and drug interactions (see package insert). *MDD*
Fluoxetine (SSRI) (Prozac®, Prozac Weekly®, Sarafem®)	For fluoxetine, Prozac: Start: 5-20 mg po q am then hold at 20 mg for 4 weeks then increase by 20 mg every 4 weeks as tolerated, stop if no improvement after 4 weeks at 60 mg/day	SSRI with longest ½ life, metabolite norfluoxetine with even longer ½ life; works a little slower than other antidepressants; inhibits CYP2C9, CYP2D6, CYP3A4. On WHO Essential Medicines List for depressive disorders. *MDD/OCD/PMDD/Bulimia /Panic Disorder*
Paroxetine (SSRI) (Paxil®, Paxil CR®)	For paroxetine, Paxil: Start: 10-20 mg po qhs and increase in 2-4 weeks to 30-40 mg/day as tolerated	SSRI most likely to cause discontinuation symptoms; SSRI most associated with treatment-emergent suicidality; produces weight gain; may have most sexual side effects; inhibits CYP2D6. *MDD/OCD/Panic Disorder/ Social anxiety disorder PTSD/GAD/PMDD*
Sertraline (SSRI) (Zoloft®)	Start: 25-50 mg po q day and maintain for 2-4 weeks, increase by 50 mg/day every 4 weeks if needed, maximum 200 mg/day but unclear if more helpful than 100 mg/day	Less enzymatic inhibition than fluoxetine, paroxetine, and fluvoxamine (although may increase lamotrigine levels); well-tolerated SSRI; may have the most favorable balance among

		benefits, side effects, and cost. *MDD/PMDD/Panic disorder* *PTSD/Social anxiety disorder* *OCD*
Fluvoxamine (SSRI) (Luvox®, Luvox CR®)	For fluvoxamine, Luvox: Start: 25 mg po bid and increase in 4 days to 100 mg/day in single or divided doses, may increase to 200 mg/day in divided dose if needed	Primarily used for OCD in U.S. due to initial application to FDA for this indication, but not likely to be more effective than other SSRIs for OCD; inhibits CYP1A2, CYP2C9, CYP2C19, CYP3A4. *OCD* *Social anxiety disorder*
Citalopram (SSRI) (Celexa®)	Start: 10-20 mg po q day and increase to 40 mg/day in 7 days, (20 mg/day may equal placebo in some studies), do not increase beyond 40 mg/day given risk of QTc prolongation at higher doses; max dose of 20 mg po q day in those with hepatic impairment or over 60 years old.	Least likely SSRI (along with escitalopram) to cause CYP450 medication interactions; well tolerated overall. Can prolong QT on doses higher than 40 mg/day. Avoid in patients who are already at higher risk of QT prolongation, or if QTc >/=500 milliseconds. Avoid use with other medications that can prolong QT. CYP2C19 substrate (avoid with other medications that may inhibit this enzyme). *Depression*
Escitalopram (SSRI) (Lexapro®)	Start: 10 mg po q day; higher doses not shown to be better but dose may be	S-citalopram; well tolerated; low risk of medication interactions;

	increased to 20 mg po q day after a minimum of 1 week.	comparison with citalopram showed about 15% better efficacy with escitalopram but this may have been an artifact of doses used. *MDD/GAD*
Venlafaxine (SNRI) (Effexor®, Effexor XR®)	For venlafaxine, Effexor: Start: 37.5 mg po q day for 4 days then increase to 75 mg daily, then add 75mg/day every week until 225 mg/day which is max for XR. Maximum is 375 mg/day for regular release venlafaxine.	Check baseline blood pressure, then every 3-6 months; an SSRI at low doses; >150 mg needed for norepinephrine effect—but increases blood pressure at these higher doses; high risk of discontinuation syndrome; low risk of enzyme inhibition; venlafaxine is still the only generic and inexpensive SNRI. *Depression/GAD/Social anxiety disorder/Panic disorder*
Duloxetine (SNRI) (Cymbalta®)	Start: 40 mg/day in single or divided doses, increase to 60 mg/day in divided doses after 3-7 days, max 120 mg/day but no evidence that increasing to maximum is more helpful.	Check baseline blood pressure, then every 3-6 months; serotonergic and noradrenergic effects at all doses; no clinically significant benefit on physical pain that often accompanies depression; avoid if substantial alcohol use or liver disease; soon to be generic; modest inhibition of CYP2D6, CYP1A2. *MDD/GAD/Diabetic peripheral neuropathy/Fibromyalgia and chronic*

		musculoskeletal pain
Bupropion (Wellbutrin®, Wellbutrin SR®, Wellbutrin XL®, ForFivo®, Zyban®)	For bupropion, Wellbutrin, Zyban: Start: 75 mg po bid or 100-150 mg q am and increase to 100-150 mg bid (2nd dose in afternoon) after 4-7 days, different dosing for different formulations	Contraindicated in patients with history of seizure, eating disorder or if otherwise at high seizure risk; least likely to cause sexual side effects or weight gain; moderate inhibition of CYP2D6. *MDD/Prevention of MDE in patients with seasonal affective disorder/Aid to smoking cessation treatment*
Mirtazapine (Remeron®)	Start: 7.5-15 mg po qhs and increase to 30 mg q hs after 4-7 days, max 45 mg po qhs	Improves appetite and sleep as early side effects; can cause weight gain; low risk of medication interactions; less sexual side effects than SSRIs; may be more sedating at lower doses; may work faster than other antidepressants. *MDD*
Trazodone (Desyrel®, Oleptro®)	For insomnia only: Start: 25 mg po qhs, if needed increase to 50 mg, then can increase by 50 mg increments up to 200 mg at bedtime. Extended release trazodone (Oleptro®): Start: 150 mg po qhs, increase by 75 mg every 4th day, maximum 375 mg po qhs.	Used primarily for insomnia; may cause orthostasis, priapism; generally not used as an antidepressant but when it was used as an antidepressant the dose was 400 mg daily; new extended release formulation is newly marketed for depression; CYP3A4 substrate. *MDD*

ANTIDEPRESSANTS

OTHER NEWER ANTIDEPRESSANTS:		
Desvenlafaxine (SNRI) (Pristiq®; Khedezla®)	Start: 50 mg po daily and continue; may go up to max of 100 mg daily but no clear benefit from doses higher than 50 mg/day.	Active metabolite of venlafaxine. Check baseline blood pressure, then every 3-6 months; high risk of discontinuation syndrome; low risk of enzyme inhibition; nausea may be early adverse effect; very expensive SNRI. CYP 3A4 substrate. *MDD*
Vilazodone (Viibryd®)	Start: 10 mg per day for first week then 20 mg per day for 2nd week, then 30 mg daily for 3rd week, then 40 mg per day; lower than 40 mg daily dose may not be effective. Take with food. Titration limited by GI symptoms.	Expensive. Unclear if with any benefits over cost-effective SSRIs and venlafaxine. Inhibits CYP2C8; CYP3A4 substrate, expected to have low drug-drug interactions. *MDD*
Isocarboxazid (MAOI) (Marplan®)	Start 10 mg po bid, if tolerated increase by 10 mg increments every 2-4 days to 40 mg po/daily total, bid to qid dosing. Max is 60 mg/day in divided doses.	Nonselective MAOI. Available for decades so not actually a 'new' MAOI but generic is now unavailable. New brand name drug is very expensive. Dangerous food and drug interactions (see package insert) *Depression*
Levomilnacipran ER (SNRI) (Fetzima®)	Start: 20 mg po daily for 2 days then increase to 40 mg po daily, then may increase in 40 mg daily increments every 2 or more days as tolerated, max is 120 mg per day. Reduce dose if renal impairment.	Check baseline blood pressure, then every 3-6 months; potent norepinephrine reuptake inhibition; CYP3A4 substrate

31

		MDD
Vortioxetine (Brintellix®)	Start: 10 mg po daily, reduce to 5 mg daily if higher doses are not tolerated, may increase to 20 mg po daily if tolerated, max is 20 mg per day.	Multiple serotonin receptor effects; nausea most common adverse effect. May displace other highly protein bound drugs; CYP2D6 substrate
		MDD

*Generic and U.S. brand name(s). **Doses are provided for educational purposes only; see package insert for dosing and other information before prescribing medications. Dosing should be adjusted downwards ('start low, go slow' strategy) for the elderly and/or the medically compromised. Abbreviations: bid-(bis in die) twice a day; CYP-Cytochrome P450 enzyme; FDA-Food and Drug Administration; GAD-Generalized Anxiety Disorder; MAOI-Monoamine Oxidase Inhibitor; MAO-B-Monoamine Oxidase Inhibitor, B subtype; MDD-Major Depressive Disorder; MDE-Major Depressive Episode; mg-milligram; ng/mL-nanogram per milliliter; OCD-Obsessive Compulsive Disorder; PMDD-Pre-menstrual Dysphoric Disorder; po-(per os) orally; PTSD-Post-traumatic Stress Disorder; q-(quaque) every; qhs-(quaque hora somni) at bedtime; SNRI-Serotonin Norepinephrine Reuptake Inhibitor; SSRI-Selective Serotonin Reuptake Inhibitor; TCA-Tricyclic Antidepressant; WHO-World Health Organization.

ANXIOLYTICS

The pharmacological treatment of anxiety symptoms is both simple and complicated. On the one hand, medications such as benzodiazepines and (now mostly obsolete) barbiturates can have a relatively immediate effect on distressing anxiety symptoms. On the other hand, the use of such medications carries the risk of cognitive impairment, physical dependence, rebound exacerbations, and the risk of psychological dependence and inappropriate use in some patients.

It is not clear that episodic anxiety that is associated with situational stressors should be treated with medications. Anxiety *per se* may be a normal response to distressing events and a signal that may enhance a person's motivation to address these real-life events. As such, it may be better understood and addressed through psychotherapy rather than pharmacologically. Students and clinicians should be aware of cultural (and managed care) pressures that push for 'popping a pill' rather than somewhat more costly counseling to improve coping strategies, much less psychotherapy, to address the underlying causes of the patient's anxiety.

Anxiety disorders are characterized by persisting patterns of anxiety symptoms impairing functioning. Examples include panic disorder, social anxiety disorder, and generalized anxiety disorder. Obsessive-compulsive disorder (OCD) and posttraumatic stress disorder (PTSD) also involve symptoms of anxiety, although they are no longer classified as anxiety disorders in the DSM-5. The first-line medication treatments for most of these anxiety-related disorders are SSRIs (or other antidepressants with serotonergic effects—these are listed in Table 1). A time period of several weeks may be necessary before clear response. During this time, anxiolytics with more immediate effects (e.g., benzodiazepines) are sometimes used for early symptom control, though their role in OCD and PTSD is more controversial.

Benzodiazepines

Benzodiazepines were first developed in the 1960s and are now the most commonly used anxiolytics in the world. **Alprazolam, lorazepam, diazepam, clonazepam, chlordiazepoxide, temazepam,** and **oxazepam** are examples of benzodiazepines. Their mechanism of action is through their binding on gamma-aminobutyric acid (GABA) receptors (Nutt and Malizia 2001). GABA is the primary inhibitory neurotransmitter in the brain. Benzodiazepines bind to one type of GABA receptor (GABAA) thereby increasing the receptor's affinity for GABA. Increased GABA effect then increases the frequency of chloride channel openings allowing this ion's influx into the cell which in turn decreases normal cell firing. The benzodiazepine binding site is composed of multiple subunits; binding to the alpha-1 subunit may explain sedative effects of benzodiazepines whereas alpha-2 subunit binding may be needed for anxiolytic effects (Nestler, Hyman, et al. 2009). In clinical practice, benzodiazepines have been used for the short-term treatment of anxiety and insomnia, as anticonvulsants, and in the treatment of alcohol withdrawal symptoms.

Benzodiazepines are associated with multiple adverse effects. They are sedating, can impair concentration, memory (Buffett-Jerrott and Stewart 2002), and coordination (e.g., as needed for motor vehicle operations), can lead to falls in the elderly (Wagner, Zhang, et al. 2004) (especially at initiation of treatment and after dose increases), and can cause respiratory depression. They are contraindicated in acute narrow or angle-closure glaucoma and may worsen glaucoma by possibly increasing intraocular pressure (Fritze, Schneider et al. 2002).

The choice of which benzodiazepine to use is often based on their pharmacokinetic properties. Diazepam, chlordiazepoxide, and clonazepam have relatively long half-lives. Diazepam and chlordiazepoxide are hepatically metabolized to desmethyldiazepam, itself a long-acting psychoactive compound. The use of these medications in hepatically compromised patients is problematic. In medically ill patients and in the elderly, benzodiazepines that do not require hepatic metabolism and have shorter half-lives such as lorazepam and oxazepam are preferred, especially when the risk of respiratory depression is a concern (e.g., patients with chronic obstructive pulmonary disease). Alprazolam has a shorter half-life than lorazepam and oxazepam. It is, however, also associated with significant rebound anxiety because of the rapid drop from peak serum level after each dose. Despite its current widespread use especially in primary care, alprazolam should generally be avoided in patients who may require frequent or daily administration of an anxiolytic drug.

Perhaps the greatest drawback of benzodiazepines, however, is that they can lead to misuse in patients with a history of alcohol or other drug use disorders. *Physical dependence* is characterized by increased tolerance to these drugs and the development of significant withdrawal symptoms upon discontinuation; this occurs with long term and/or high dose use of benzodiazepines and is not necessarily a sign of misuse (although patients should be made aware of the need for very gradual taper of these medications if used long term). A *benzodiazepine use disorder*, on the other hand, is characterized by maladaptive behavioral changes leading to medication misuse. Benzodiazepines (along with barbiturates discussed below) are controlled substances which should be prescribed judiciously and cautiously and only when adequate follow-up is available to ensure appropriate use. It should be noted that adequate follow-up is not often feasible in some primary care settings. Benzodiazepines should generally be avoided in any patient with a history of a substance or alcohol use disorder: as noted, most benzodiazepine misuse occurs in these individuals. There are circumstances in which a patient with a history of substance abuse may require benzodiazepines (for example a patient with a severe debilitating panic disorder who has been refractory to all other non-benzodiazepine medications)—these circumstances, however, should be considered infrequent (Osser, Renner, Bayog 1999).

Barbiturates

Discovered more than 100 years ago and developed in the 1940's and 50's, barbiturates are now rarely used for the treatment of anxiety due to a higher risk of dependence and dangerousness in overdose when compared to benzodiazepines. Whereas benzodiazepine binding increases the receptor's affinity for GABA and indirectly affects chloride channels, barbiturates (and alcohol), binding on a different site on GABAA receptors, can increase chloride influx into neurons even when GABA is not present (Loscher and Rogawski 2012). **Chloral hydrate**, a weaker barbiturate but with the same risks, is still occasionally used in certain settings for the treatment of refractory insomnia or for sedation prior to anxiety provoking medical studies (e.g., MRI). Other barbiturates such as **phenobarbital, pentobarbital,** and **butalbital,** are still occasionally used for treatment of conditions (e.g., seizure disorder, migraine) other than anxiety disorders.

Medicines without Abuse Potential Used for the Treatment of Anxiety

Buspirone is a 5HT1A receptor partial agonist (primarily, but not exclusively, on presynaptic autoreceptors) that may affect serotonin release from serotonergic neurons. Buspirone has no effect on GABA receptors and as such cannot immediately replace benzodiazepines. It has no immediate anxiolytic effects. However, it has no potential for abuse, and does not impair cognition or motor coordination. Side effects, however, may include headache, insomnia, jitteriness and nausea. It is efficacious for the treatment of generalized anxiety disorder.

Propranolol is a beta-adrenergic antagonist. Although it is primarily used medically for its effect on heart rate and blood pressure, its 'off-label' use in psychiatry is based on its ability to reduce overall sympathetic activation. It is particularly helpful in circumstances where a sympathetic reaction to an anxiety-provoking stimulus can occur, such as in instances of performance anxiety. Musicians, for example, may take a dose one hour prior to their appearance on stage, where it may decrease somatic manifestations of anxiety such as tremulousness and tachycardia. It does not, however, help alleviate symptoms associated with generalized social phobia or generalized anxiety disorder. Propranolol should be avoided if the patient has congestive heart failure or significant asthma. Despite earlier concerns that beta-blockers may cause depression (Waal 1967) this is not supported by more recent studies (Ko, Hebert, et al. 2002).

Clonidine, initially developed as an antihypertensive, is an alpha-2-adrenergic autoreceptor agonist which serves to decrease sympathetic drive in the locus ceruleus. Uncontrolled reports suggest it can decrease hyperarousal in patients with posttraumatic stress disorder (Boehnlein and Kinzie 2007) and other conditions associated with autonomic hyperactivity (e.g. rebound hyperactivity in opioid withdrawal states).

Prazosin is an alpha-1-adrenergic receptor antagonist. Like clonidine, it is an antihypertensive which seems to decrease anxiety symptoms and insomnia associated with posttraumatic states. It has no sedative properties but it can help decrease PTSD symptoms during the day and decrease nightmares and disturbed awakenings at night (Taylor, Lowe, et al. 2006; Raskind, Peskind, et al. 2007; Miller 2008; Taylor, Martin, et al. 2008). Newer studies have added to the evidence supporting the efficacy of prazosin in the treatment of PTSD-related nightmares, hyperarousal, and insomnia, while being generally well-tolerated despite the possibility of lowering blood pressure (Byers, Allison et al. 2010; Calohan, Peterson et al. 2010; Germain, Richardson et al. 2012; Hudson, Whiteside et al. 2012; Kung, Espinel et al. 2012; Raskind, Peterson et al. 2013). Some have called prazosin the 'penicillin for PTSD' because it works so well in many patients. However, it requires slow titration, to minimize the risk of hypotension, from 1 mg at bedtime up to a mean dose of 16 mg in some male veterans with PTSD (Raskind, Peterson et al. 2013). This usually takes weeks so some clinicians will try clonidine instead despite its minimal evidence-base.

Hydroxyzine is an antihistamine with less affinity for muscarinic and alpha-1-adrenergic receptors than other antihistamines. Because it does not cause dependence and has no abuse potential, it is useful for treating anxiety symptoms in patients with a history of substance use disorders. Available since the 1950s, hydroxy-zine's role in the treatment of anxiety was initially overshadowed by the newer benzodiazepines. Currently however it has had a reemergence as a versatile drug in the psychiatric armamentarium (Dowben, Grant et al. 2013). It has been shown to have efficacy in the treatment of generalized anxiety disorder (Ferreri, and Hantouche, et al. 1994; Darcis 1995; Lader and Scotto 1998; Llorca, Spadone, et al. 2002; Guaiana, Barbui et al. 2010). Also, it is frequently used (particularly as an 'as needed' medication on inpatient settings) for the treatment of anxiety and insomnia in patients for whom other anxiolytics or sedating medications (e.g. benzodiazepines or sedating antipsychotics) are undesirable. Hydroxyzine's antihistaminic, antiemetic, and possible (but not confirmed) pain-reducing potentiation effects can render it very useful for many patients with comorbid anxiety.

Newer Hypnotics

Zolpidem, zaleplon, and **eszopiclone** (enantiomer of zopiclone, a hypnotic not available in the U.S.) are non-benzodiazepine hypnotics that bind to alpha-1 subunits on the benzodiazepine binding site on GABA receptors (Sanger 2004). These 'z-drugs' cause sedation but lack anxiolytic effects despite some cross-reactivity with benzodiazepines. Although their abuse potential is purportedly less than benzodiazepines, they are not free from the risk of dependence and withdrawal symptoms upon discontinuation (Liappas, Malitas, et al. 2003; Sethi and Khandelwal 2005; Cubala and Landowski 2007; Victorri-Vigneau, Dailly, et al. 2007). There is insufficient evidence that these hypnotics are either more effective or safer than benzodiazepines—for example, zolpidem increased the risk for hip fractures up to 2-fold in patients over 65 years old after controlling for multiple possible covariates (Lin, Chen et al. 2014). However, successful marketing has resulted in widespread use when more cost-effective treatments could have been considered (Glass, Lanctot, et al. 2005; Siriwardena, Qureshi, et al. 2006). Zolpidem is now generic, but zaleplon and eszopiclone are still brand products and are expensive. A recent review of FDA data suggests that although non-benzodiazepine hypnotics may reduce sleep latency, their effects on polysomnographic sleep latency and subjective sleep latency are relatively small (Huedo-Medina, Kirsch et al. 2012).

Ramelteon is a fairly new hypnotic that is an MT1 and MT2 melatonin receptor agonist which may have modest efficacy in shortening sleep latency but not in increasing total sleep duration (Roth, Seiden, et al. 2006; Sateia, Kirby-Long, et al. 2008; Liu and Wang 2012). It is well-tolerated (Johnson, Suess, et al. 2006; Mets, van Deventer et al. 2010) but again there are no studies to suggest it should be favored over more cost-effective alternatives.

Suvorexant, an orexin receptor antagonist, is the latest drug to be approved by the FDA for the treatment of insomnia. Orexins are neuropeptides secreted by the neurons of the hypothalamus that act to regulate wakefulness and arousal; an antagonist at orexin receptors would therefore likely inhibit wakefulness and facilitate sleep (Ebrahim, Howard et al. 2002; Bennett, Bray et al. 2014). Suvorexant is not available for sale in the U.S. at the time of this writing and there is as of yet insufficient clinical experience to support its use. Next day residual sedative effects may be a risk at higher doses (Sun, Kennedy et al. 2013).

When considering treatment of chronic insomnia, prescribing clinicians should thoroughly review the differential diagnosis of possible contributing factors (Schutte-Rodin, Broch et al. 2008), and not overlook the benefits that may be derived from nonpharmacological, e.g., behavioral, therapies (Sivertsen, Omvik, et al. 2006).

Further Notes on the Use of Benzodiazepines and 'Z-Drugs'

Benzodiazepines: Despite their many potential risks, benzodiazepines continue to be commonly prescribed for the treatment of anxiety and insomnia. Because they are highly effective in relieving short-term anxiety, they are often continued either due to patient request or because the prescribing clinician does not believe that adequately effective alternative medications are available. However as noted in this chapter, effective alternatives do exist for the treatment of most anxiety disorders and these should be considered. When benzodiazepines (or 'z-drugs') are continued over the long run, short-term adverse risks are perpetuated and possibly even compounded over time. Many of these short-term risks have already been discussed above. The following considerations should also be taken into account:

1. As previously noted, the use of benzodiazepines can increase the risk of falls, especially in the elderly. A recent review of the association between benzodiazepine use and hip fractures across five Western European countries and the United States showed that an estimated 1.8-8.2% of hip fractures may be attributable to benzodiazepine use, with variations based on differences in benzodiazepine use in these countries (Khong, de Vries et al. 2012). Short-acting benzodiazepines appeared to be associated with hip fractures more than long-acting benzodiazepines (although other studies have found a greater association with the latter). In another large study of older VA outpatients, the number of inpatient and outpatient treatment encounters for physical 'injuries' was significantly increased in outpatient benzodiazepine users when compared with the controlled cohort (French, Spehar et al. 2005).

2. Memory and cognitive impairments that can occur with short-term use are also seen with long-term use. A review of literature studying long-term benzodiazepines users (mean of 9.9 years) found evidence of significant cognitive impairment across multiple domains (such as information processing, memory and attention) when compared to controls, with some indication that impairment may worsen with increased duration of use (Barker, Greenwood et al. 2004). A recent study of young adults also confirmed an association between long-term use of benzodiazepines and impairment in long-term memory in women (Boeuf-Cazou, Bongue et al. 2011). Long-term impairments may not subside entirely after benzodiazepine discontinuation (Barker, Greenwood et al. 2004).

3. Exposure to benzodiazepines appears to increase the risk of traffic accidents. The risk appears higher with the use of long-acting benzodiazepines, at initiation of use, and with higher doses (Smink, Egberts et al. 2010). As expected, in drivers who are found to be impaired and have a positive toxicology screen for benzodiazepines, the degree of impairment directly correlates with the benzodiazepine blood level (Bramness, Skurtveit et al. 2002).

4. The combination of benzodiazepines with other hypnotics, barbiturates, and opiates carries higher risks than those associated with each of these substances alone. The adverse physical, psychological and cognitive effects that have been discussed above can also be significantly compounded—e.g., possibly even to lethal levels as in the case of the increased risk of respiratory depression. The risk of physical injury can also significantly

increase (French, Chirikos et al. 2005). Although some patients may combine benzodiazepines with other substances, such as opiates, to enhance the expected euphoria (Jones, Mogali et al. 2012), for many patients the combination of medications begins as an honest effort by their prescribing clinician to treat the various presenting symptoms. Unfortunately, it is not rare to see a patient who has been concurrently prescribed a daily benzodiazepine for anxiety, zolpidem for insomnia, an opiate for pain, and a migraine medication that includes butalbital (*and* who may choose to add a daily glass or more of wine to the mix), who then continues this regimen over the long term. Even if all these medications are taken 'as prescribed,' the risks for dangerous events to occur (as has been seen in certain celebrities recently) is very high. An appropriate role of the psychiatric clinician can be to attempt to help the patient and the primary prescribing clinician gradually lower the overall medication load and to explore factors that have may have led to this polypharmacy.

Given the above concerns, efforts should be made to limit benzodiazepines to short-term use whenever possible. Those who have been on long-term treatment and are not doing well should be considered for tapering and replacement of these medications. Gradual dose reduction, in combination with psychological treatments, appears effective in helping patients discontinue benzodiazepine use (Parr, Kavanagh et al. 2009). Surprisingly, simple and 'minimal' interventions such as a single letter sent from a family physician recommending dose reduction or discontinuation has been shown to considerably reduce long-term use of benzodiazepines in some patients (Gorgels, Oude Voshaar et al. 2005; Mugunthan, McGuire et al. 2011). Additionally, in one study, the majority of patients who had stopped use after receiving a discontinuation letter from their general practitioner were not using benzodiazepines at 10-year follow up. Clearly, given the evidence, there is a likelihood of succeeding in decreasing overall risk and side effect burden if clinicians placed a stronger emphasis on reducing long-term benzodiazepine use in their patients.

'Z-Drugs': More recently, multiple additional concerns have been raised about the safety of these hypnotics (especially about the safety of zolpidem for which there are more available data). Although many of these concerns and risks may also apply to benzodiazepines, increasingly both medical and behavioral side effects of non-benzodiazepines hypnotics have been reported:

1. Zolpidem use can significantly increase falls in inpatients settings. Patients who were treated with zolpidem had an over 4-fold increase in falls compared to those who were prescribed the drug but did not take it (Kolla, Lovely et al. 2013).

2. The FDA issued warnings in 2013 that the use of higher doses of zolpidem "can increase the risk of next-day impairment of driving and other activities that require full alertness" and suggested a lowering of recommended doses especially in women. It also warned that when taking extended-release zolpidem patients "should not drive or engage in other activities that require complete mental alertness the day after taking the drug because zolpidem levels can remain high enough the next

day to impair these activities" (FDA 2013; PDR 2014). The use of 'z-drugs' (as well as benzodiazepines) has been associated with an increase in road traffic accidents (Gustavsen, Bramness et al. 2008; Orriols, Philip et al. 2011).

3. Sleep-related behavioral changes have been observed after taking 'z-drugs' (mostly zolpidem) for sleep (Logan and Couper 2001; Morgenthaler and Silber 2002; Doane and Dalpiaz 2008; Dolder and Nelson 2008). These behaviors could include, but are not limited to, sleep-walking, sleep-eating, sleep-conversations, and sleep-driving. Although these are considered to be rare side effects, one small retrospective study found that slightly over 5% of patients taking zolpidem reported changes in sleep-related behaviors (Tsai, Yang et al. 2009). The occurrence of these behaviors is likely to be underreported given that the behaviors are usually accompanied by amnesia.

Given the above, before prescribing non-benzodiazepine hypnotics, clinicians should ask themselves if the proposed medication offers any benefits over other available agents (and non-psychopharmacological interventions) that may be helpful for the causes of the insomnia. Risks and benefits should be discussed with patients. The underlying causes of the insomnia should always be identified: often there is a psychiatric or medical disorder that requires treatment other than a benzodiazepine or z-drug. Furthermore, if a benzodiazepine or non-benzodiazepine hypnotic is chosen, the goal should remain to use the medication for the short-term only.

Table of Anxiolytics and Hypnotics

Table 2 summarizes the characteristics of selected non-antidepressant medications for the treatment of anxiety and insomnia (Ansari and Osser 2009; WHO 2011; PDR 2014). Antidepressants used in the treatment of anxiety disorders are listed in Table 1.

TABLE 2. SELECTED NON-ANTIDEPRESSANT MEDICATIONS FOR ANXIETY AND INSOMNIA

MEDICATION*	DOSING**	COMMENTS/ *FDA Indication*
Clonazepam (Benzodiazepine) (Klonopin®, Clonazepam Orally Disintegrating Tablets®)	Start: 0.25-0.5 mg po bid for panic disorder. increase as needed, use lowest effective dose. Equivalence: 0.25 mg equals lorazepam 1 mg. Tmax = 1-4 hrs t ½ = 30-50 hrs	Benzodiazepine with convenient pharmacokinetics for the treatment of panic disorder (30-50 hours half-life); has treatment-emergent suicide risk warning in package insert as do all antiepileptic drugs; CYP3A4 substrate. *Panic disorder/Specific seizure disorders (see package insert)*
Diazepam (Benzodiazepine) (Valium®, Diastat®, Diazepam Injection®)	For oral diazepam, Valium: Start: 2 mg po bid-tid, increase as needed, use lowest effective dose. Equivalence: 5 mg equals lorazepam 1 mg. Tmax = 1-1.5 hrs t ½ = 48-100 hrs (if including t ½ of active metabolite).	Rapid onset of action due to lipid solubility followed by rapid distribution to lipid compartment, long elimination half-life because of metabolite. On WHO Essential Medicines List for generalized anxiety and sleep disorders, and as an anticonvulsant. *Anxiety disorders and short-term relief of anxiety symptoms/Acute alcohol withdrawal symptoms/Adjunctive treatment for convulsive disorders/Adjunctive therapy in skeletal muscle spasms*
Chlordiazepoxide (Benzodiazepine) (Librium®)	Start: 10 mg po tid-qid, increase as needed, use lowest effective dose. Equivalence: 25 mg equals lorazepam 1 mg.	Frequently used in inpatient detoxification for severe alcohol withdrawal symptoms when there is no hepatic dysfunction; multiple psychoactive metabolites.

	Tmax = 1-4 hrs t ½ = 48-100 hrs (if including t ½ of active metabolite)	*Anxiety disorders and short-term relief of anxiety symptoms/Acute alcohol withdrawal symptoms/Preoperative anxiety and apprehension*
Oxazepam (Benzodiazepine) (Serax®)	Start: 10 mg po tid, increase as needed, use lowest effective dose. Equivalence: 15 mg equals lorazepam 1 mg. Tmax = 3 hrs (5 hours in elderly, so not practical as a 'prn') t ½ = 8 hrs	Used in inpatient detoxification when hepatic impairment is present; slowest onset of action among benzodiazepines. *Anxiety disorders and short-term relief of anxiety symptoms/Anxiety associated with depression/Management of anxiety in the elderly/Acute alcohol withdrawal*
Lorazepam (Benzodiazepine) (Ativan®, Ativan Injection®)	For oral lorazepam, Ativan: Start: 0.5 mg po bid-tid, increase as needed, use lowest effective dose. Tmax = 2 hrs t ½ = 12 hrs	Most widely used in inpatient setting for 'as needed' treatment of anxiety, agitation, and withdrawal states; only benzodiazepine available IM (except for diazepam which is available but not reliably absorbed IM). *Anxiety disorders and short-term relief of anxiety symptoms or anxiety associated with depressive symptoms/Status epilepticus (for injection)/Preanesthetic medication for adults (for injection)*
Alprazolam (Benzodiazepine) (Xanax®, Xanax XR®,	For alprazolam, Xanax, Niravam:	Most addictive benzodiazepine—greatest

Niravam®)	Usual starting dose is 0.25 mg po tid, change to other benzodiazepine if ongoing treatment is needed. Equivalence: 0.5 mg equals lorazepam 1 mg. Tmax = 1-2 hrs t ½ = 6-11 hrs	euphoric effect in alcoholic patients; infrequent 'as needed' use may be appropriate; CYP3A4 substrate. *Anxiety disorders and short-term relief of anxiety symptoms/Panic disorder*
Buspirone (Atypical anxiolytic—5HT1A partial agonist) (Buspar®)	Start: 5 mg po bid-tid; increase every 2-3 days by 5-10 mg to 30-40 mg in two divided doses, maximum dose is 60 mg/day.	Alcoholics with anxiety may require near maximum doses; use for symptoms corresponding to generalized anxiety disorder (not helpful with short-term relief of anxiety symptoms despite FDA indication below); CYP3A4 substrate. *Anxiety disorders and short-term relief of anxiety symptoms*
Propranolol (Beta-blocker) (Inderal®, Inderal LA®, Innopran XL®)	For propranolol, Inderal: Start: test dose of 10 mg po, then gradually up to 40 mg 30-60 minutes before anxiety provoking event.	Also used in psychiatry to treat akathisia, lithium-induced tremor, and clozapine-induced tachycardia. When taken daily requires gradual taper if stopping use, given cardiac risks upon abrupt discontinuation. *Migraine prophylaxis/ Hypertension/Other cardiac conditions (see package*

ANXIOLYTICS

		insert)
Clonidine (Antihypertensive— Alpha 2 agonist) (Catapres®, Catapres-TTS®)	For oral clonidine, Catapres: Start: 0.1 mg po bid or qhs, increase as needed and tolerated	May be helpful for hyperarousal associated with PTSD. Also used for opiate withdrawal.
		Hypertension
Prazosin (Antihypertensive— Alpha 1 antagonist) (Minipress®)	Starting dose for males: 1 mg po qhs, after 2 days increase to 2 mg po qhs, after 5 more days increase to 4 mg po qhs, if no response after 7 days then increase to 6 mg po qhs, after another 7 days increase to 10 mg po qhs, then to 15 mg po qhs after another 7 days, then to 20 mg po qhs. Dosage for women is lower, with max of 10 mg po qhs	Helpful for insomnia, nightmares, and disturbed awakenings associated with PTSD. Also can be titrated gradually up to 5 mg daily for daytime PTSD symptoms in men and 2 mg daily for women.
		Hypertension
Hydroxyzine (Antihistamine— H1 antagonist) (Atarax®, Vistaril®)	Start: 10-12.5 mg po morning and midday and 20-25 mg po qhs for generalized anxiety disorder. Anecdotal usage at higher doses.	May also have analgesic effects; muscle relaxation properties, bronchodilator activity, antiemetic, antihistamine, may help with insomnia.
		Anxiety symptoms/Multiple

		other indications(see package insert)
Zolpidem (Hypnotic) (Ambien®, Ambien-CR®, Edluar®, Intermezzo®, ZolpiMist® (mouth spray))	For zolpidem, Ambien: Start: 5 mg po qhs, may increase to 10 mg po qhs if needed but be aware of risk of next day impairment; (see package insert for other formulations). Tmax = 1.6 hrs t ½ = 2-3 hrs	Rapid onset; reported cases of amnesia; sertraline may increase serum level. FDA alert in 2013 recommending lower nightly doses to decrease risk of next day impairment with increased risk of impairment seen in women and with Ambien-CR. FDA also warns that patients taking Ambien-CR at night should not drive the next morning. *Short-term treatment of insomnia characterized by difficulties with sleep initiation*
Zaleplon (Hypnotic) (Sonata®)	Start: 5 mg po qhs, may increase to 10 mg qhs, maximum 20 mg po qhs. Tmax = 1 hour t ½ = 1 hour	Amnesia may occur as it does with benzodiazepines; ultra-short half-life; expensive; CYP3A4 substrate. *Short-term treatment of insomnia*
Eszopiclone (Hypnotic) (Lunesta®)	Start: 1-2 mg po qhs, maximum 3 mg po qhs. Tmax = 1 hour t ½ = 6 hours	Amnesia may occur; similar dependence potential and A.M. driving impairment to diazepam; expensive with no advantages; CYP3A4 substrate. *Treatment of insomnia*
Ramelteon (Melatonin receptor agonist) (Rozerem®)	8 mg po within 30 minutes of bedtime, do not take with fatty meal. Tmax = 0.75 hrs	No DEA restriction; very short half-life; expensive; Unclear if any different in effect from over the counter melatonin. CYP1A2, CYP2C9, and CYP3A4

	t ½ = 1.5 hrs	substrate.
		Treatment of insomnia characterized by difficulty with sleep onset

*Generic and U.S. brand name(s). ** Doses are provided for educational purposes only; see package insert for dosing and other information before prescribing medications. Dosing should be adjusted downwards ('start low, go slow' strategy) for the elderly and/or the medically compromised. Abbreviations: bid-(bis in die) twice a day; CYP-Cytochrome P450 enzyme; DEA-Drug Enforcement Administration; FDA-Food and Drug Administration; IM-intramuscular; mg-milligram; po-(per os) orally; PTSD-Posttraumatic Stress Disorder; qhs-(quaque hora somni) at bedtime; qid-(quater in die) four times a day; tid-(ter in die) three times a day; Tmax-time from administration to maximum serum concentration; t ½ -medication half-life; WHO-World Health Organization.

ANTIPSYCHOTICS

First Generation Antipsychotics

The first antipsychotic, chlorpromazine, was developed in the 1950s (Meyer and Simpson 1997). Subsequently other antipsychotics were developed that share similarities in their mechanisms of action and in their side effect profiles. **Chlorpromazine, thioridazine, perphenazine, thiothixene, pimozide, fluphenazine,** and **haloperidol** are examples of these medications that are now characterized as 'first generation antipsychotics' (FGAs). Alternative names for this class of medications include: 'neuroleptics' (for their propensity to cause adverse neurological effects), 'major tranquilizers' (as opposed to the later designated 'minor tranquilizers' such as benzodiazepines and barbiturates), 'typical' antipsychotics (because of their ability to cause typical parkinsonian side effects), and 'conventional' antipsychotics.

All first generation antipsychotics are believed to exert their antipsychotic effects through post-synaptic D2 dopamine receptor antagonism, thereby reducing the effect of endogenous dopamine released by presynaptic dopaminergic neurons (Nestler, Hyman, et al. 2009). In doing so, they bind more tightly to the D2 receptor than dopamine itself (Seeman 2002).

Dopaminergic neurons originate from 3 distinct nuclei. One group of dopaminergic neurons projects from the ventral tegmental area of the midbrain to the nucleus accumbens, cingulate cortex and prefrontal cortex (the mesolimbic and mesocortical tracks); these affect emotions and cognition and as such are the targets for the therapeutic effects of antipsychotic drugs. Dopaminergic neurons also arise from the substantia nigra and project to the striatum (the nigrostriatal track); these are implicated in the neurological side effects of antipsychotics. And finally, hypothalamic dopaminergic neurons project to the pituitary gland and serve to regulate the release of prolactin (the tuberoinfundibular track); disruption of this system with D2 blockade can result in hyperprolactinemia associated with the use of antipsychotics. Overall, in terms of clinical use, it has been shown that the optimal D2 receptor occupancy level for maximizing antipsychotic effect while minimizing adverse effects is 60-70% (Farde, Nordstrom, et al. 1992). The D2 receptor occupancy level for eliciting extrapyramidal (neuroleptic) symptoms is about 80% (Seeman 2002).

FGAs have traditionally been divided into low potency (e.g., chlorpromazine, thioridazine), mid-potency (e.g., perphenazine, thiothixene), and high potency (e.g., haloperidol, fluphenazine) antipsychotics, based on the number of milligrams of each drug needed to show comparable efficacy. For example, chlorpromazine 300 mg (low potency) may have the same therapeutic effect as perphenazine 24 mg (mid-potency) and haloperidol 6 mg (high potency). FGAs are often listed as a spectrum from low to high potency. The low potency antipsychotics usually exhibit tricyclic antidepressant (TCA)-like side effects such as anticholinergic, antihistaminic, and orthostatic effects (see section on antidepressants) but have a lower risk of causing acute neurological side effects such as acute muscle dystonias. At the other end of the spectrum, high potency FGAs have lower risks of TCA-like adverse effects but a much higher risk of causing acute dystonias. Mid-potency antipsychotics share all these side effects but less so than those of either pole. Clinicians today use the FGAs less often; still they should become familiar with using at least one antipsychotic from each potency class in order to be able to match the side effect profile to the patient's pre-existing vulnerabilities.

When dosing FGAs, it is important to consider that although in most efficacy studies the presumed therapeutic dose of haloperidol is 10 mg/day or more, the ideal dose may be much lower: haloperidol 2 mg/day in neuroleptic-naïve patients, and 4 mg in non-neuroleptic-naïve patients may be sufficient to produce a 'neuroleptic threshold'—the dose at which cogwheel rigidity, a sign of more-than-sufficient D2 receptor blockade, first appears (McEvoy, Stiller, et al. 1986).

The propensity of FGAs to cause neurological symptoms such as acute muscle dystonias, parkinsonism, akathisia, and tardive dyskinesia significantly limits their use in current practice. *Acute dystonias*, which are more likely to occur if the patient is young, male, has a history of substance abuse and/or a prior history of dystonias, are primarily seen in patients taking FGAs, although they can also occur in patients on any antipsychotic with significant D2 receptor antagonism (see risperidone below). Use of anticholinergic medications, such as benztropine or diphenhydramine (or promethazine used more often outside the U.S.) can decrease the occurrence of early dystonias, or treat them acutely. *Parkinsonism*, characterized by bradykinesia, tremor, rigidity, and masked facies, can develop after 1-4 weeks of treatment with FGAs. Anticholinergic medications or a dopamine releasing agent such as amantadine may be helpful, although changing the antipsychotic may be required. *Akathisia*, which is an unpleasant subjective sense of inner restlessness relieved by movement, is also commonly seen in patients treated with FGAs. Identifying akathisia as a cause of agitation (or even worsening psychosis or suicidality) is important because treatment would include decreasing, rather than increasing, the antipsychotic dose. Akathisia is treated with beta-blockers, benzodiazepines, and anticholinergic agents. *Tardive dyskinesia* (TD), a potentially irreversible syndrome of abnormal involuntary movements, can develop with extended use of antipsychotics, especially if high doses are used for long periods of time. Patients with prolonged antipsychotic treatment, a history of affective disorders, a history of parkinsonian side effects with initial antipsychotic treatment, as well as women and the elderly, are at a higher risk for developing TD. Once tardive dyskinesia has developed, withdrawal of the antipsychotic (especially if this is precipitous) may unmask worsened abnormal movements. Resumption of antipsychotic treatment may suppress these symptoms for a period of time, but progression of the underlying movement disorder toward permanence may continue.

Despite trials of multiple remedies, treatments for TD are generally only partially effective (Soares-Weiser and Fernandez 2007). In clinical settings, treatments that are usually considered include antipsychotic dose reduction or switching to a second generation antipsychotic (especially clozapine—see below) (van Harten and Tenback 2011). Daily supplementation with Vitamin E, which has been frequently proposed as first-line for treating TD, may not improve involuntary movements once they have been established (although concomitant use may protect against worsening TD) (Soares-Weiser, Maayan et al. 2011). Data from small trials and case reports suggest that deep brain stimulation may help improve TD (Mentzel, Tenback et al. 2012). Other remedies with some evidence of efficacy include vitamin B6, donepezil, and melatonin (Lerner, Miodownik et al. 2001; Caroff, Campbell et al. 2001; Shamir, Barak et al. 2001).

Neuroleptic malignant syndrome (NMS) is a poorly understood, rare, but potentially fatal complication of treatment with FGAs and other antipsychotics. NMS is characterized by a constellation of symptoms that may include delirium, lead-pipe rigidity, autonomic instability and high fevers. It can develop very early in the course of antipsychotic treatment. A high serum creatine phosphokinase (CPK) and elevated white blood cell count are supportive of the diagnosis of NMS. If NMS appears likely then the offending antipsychotic should be immediately discontinued. Medical hospitalization is necessary and treatment may include the use of a dopamine agonist (e.g., bromocriptine), a muscle relaxant (e.g., dantrolene), aggressive hydration, and the use of benzodiazepines if needed for behavioral agitation (Hu and Frucht 2007). Once the patient has been medically stabilized, the offending agent should be avoided. Rechallenge with another antipsychotic may be possible two weeks after all symptoms of NMS have abated, optimally with a low potency agent.

Second Generation Antipsychotics

Second generation antipsychotics (SGAs), also known as atypical antipsychotics, are believed to exert their antipsychotic effects through a similar mechanism of action (i.e., dopamine antagonism), but have profiles of receptor activity that produce different side effects than FGAs. Although their antipsychotic effect is believed to be due to D2 receptor antagonism, most SGAs, in contrast to FGAs, bind less tightly to these receptors than dopamine (Seeman 2002); they also more rapidly dissociate from the D2 receptors (Stahl 2001). SGAs also bind to 5HT2A serotonin receptors which may have some effect in indirectly reducing their neuroleptic risks (but not their antipsychotic effects) (Stahl 2001). The first SGA to be developed was **clozapine**, which was followed by the sequential introduction of **risperidone, olanzapine, quetiapine, ziprasidone,** and **aripiprazole** in the United States (and amisulpride and zotepine among others, in other countries). Recently four newer SGAs, namely **paliperidone, iloperidone, asenapine,** and **lurasidone** have also been introduced in the U.S. Whereas FGAs were known to (1) possibly worsen (or at least not improve) the negative symptoms of schizophrenia and (2) cause extrapyramidal symptoms including TD, SGAs were hoped to be more effective in treating negative symptoms and less likely to cause movement disorders. It is true that, by and large, SGAs do not worsen negative symptoms of schizophrenia and have a much lower risk of causing TD (Correll, Leucht, et al. 2004; Tarsy, Lungu et al. 2011). Although most EPS symptoms are relatively uncommon with SGAs (except in high doses), akathisia is common with some. NMS can rarely occur with SGAs, and may present similarly as in FGAs (although it may present differently with the atypical clozapine, discussed below, where it may exhibit with less muscle rigidity) (Trollor, Chen et al. 2009).

Questions, however, regarding the differential effectiveness of SGAs as compared with FGAs, and the SGAs' greater risks of inducing other, non-neurological, adverse effects have served to dampen the optimistic expectations initially associated with these newer medications. Nevertheless, in most of the world where they are available, SGAs are still considered to be the first-line for treatment of psychotic disorders primarily because of the reduced risk of TD.

Risperidone, one of the earliest SGAs to be developed, was released in 1994. It is similar to FGAs in that it is a potent D2 receptor antagonist, but like many other SGAs, it is also a post-synaptic serotonin 5HT2A antagonist. This is thought to mitigate the D2 receptor-mediated neurological side effects. Because of its D2 blocking potency, it is likely to have a higher risk of causing EPS and hyperprolactinemia than other SGAs (except for paliperidone—see below) (Komossa, Rummel-Kluge et al. 2011). Nevertheless, at doses lower than 6 mg/day (i.e., at usual therapeutic doses), risperidone carries a low risk of causing EPS; at higher doses, D2 blockade effects predominate and the risk of EPS increases significantly. EPS are usually not present at risperidone 3 mg/day—a dose at which 72% of D2 receptors are occupied (Nyberg, Eriksson, et al. 1999). The optimal dose derived from clinical studies appears to be 3-6 mg daily (Osser and Sigadel 2001). Although generally a well-tolerated antipsychotic, other side effects of risperidone include possible hypotension, and in children and adolescents it produces considerable weight gain (Sikich, Frazier, et al. 2008). It is a hepatic CYP2D6 enzyme substrate and therefore its metabolism can be slowed by (1) inhibitors such as fluoxetine and paroxetine (Spina, Scordo, et al. 2003), or (2) the CYP2D6 variant gene for slow metabolism, which results in a less active form of the CYP2D6 enzyme (found more often in Chinese and other East Asian individuals) (Bertilsson 1995). Another gene variant that causes "poor" metabolism is more common in Caucasians and results in severe side effects. Risperidone has a medium propensity to cause adverse metabolic effects in adults (see discussion below). On the positive side, it may have a somewhat more rapid onset of action compared to other second generation antipsychotics (Osser and Sigadel 2001).

Olanzapine was introduced in 1996. It has less affinity for D2 receptors than risperidone and a greater affinity for 5HT2A and 5HT2C serotonin receptors. Olanzapine also has significant antihistaminic and anticholinergic effects. Although it is an effective antipsychotic for the treatment of schizophrenia (Komossa, Rummel-Kluge et al. 2010) (especially at doses equal to or greater than 15 mg/day) (Osser and Sigadel 2001), it is (along with clozapine as discussed below) a frequent cause of weight gain, insulin resistance, and hyperlipidemia (i.e., 'metabolic syndrome'). Concern about the increased morbidity and mortality associated with the metabolic syndrome has lead to a reduction of the use of olanzapine in recent years. Many practice guidelines have proposed that it be avoided as a first-line agent because of these adverse effects (Osser, Roudsari et al. 2013; Mohammad and Osser 2014). All side effects increase when olanzapine is used at higher than recommended doses (e.g., 40 mg/day vs. the package insert maximum dose of 20 mg/day) with no additional antipsychotic benefit (Kinon, Volavka et al. 2008; Citrom, Stauffer et al. 2009; Osser, Roudsari et al. 2013). Liver transaminases can also become transiently elevated more often with olanzapine than with risperidone.

Quetiapine shows weak binding affinity at both dopamine and 5HT2 serotonin receptors, but with overall similar receptor occupancy to the more potent SGAs (Seeman 2002). It has alpha-adrenergic antagonism and antihistaminic effects, causing orthostasis and sedation, respectively. Quetiapine is less likely than olanzapine and clozapine, but more likely than most FGAs, risperidone and other SGAs, to cause metabolic side effects. Quetiapine at low doses, which may still be associated with weight gain (Williams, Alinejad et al. 2010), is widely (and too readily) used in psychiatric practice for the treatment of insomnia and acute anxiety in a wide range of patients with personality and/or substance abuse disorders for whom benzodiazepine use may be problematic. This 'off-label' use should only be considered after a thoughtful review of risks, benefits, and alternative treatments, especially evidence-supported treatments, for the patient's diagnosed condition. Clinicians should be aware also of reports of abuse and 'street value' for this medication (Hanley and Kenna 2008). Use of quetiapine for anxiety symptoms may be more appropriate in acute care settings such as during hospitalizations. Quetiapine's effectiveness in psychotic disorders may be less than that of olanzapine and risperidone (McCue, Waheed, et al. 2006; Suzuki, Uchida, et al. 2007), and it has among the lowest success rates in preventing future episodes (Kreyenbuhl, Slade et al. 2011). Using quetiapine at doses higher than usual approved doses (i.e., greater than 800 mg/day) does not appear to provide any added benefit and is not recommended (Lindenmayer, Citrome et al. 2011; Honer, MacEwan et al. 2012). Quetiapine produces significant QTc prolongation and a package insert warning added in 2011 cites 12 medications with which it should not be combined. Quetiapine may have a stronger role in treating patients with bipolar disorders (see chapter on mood stabilizers).

Ziprasidone is an SGA with moderate D2 antagonism and significant 5HT2A antagonism (i.e.. a high 5HT2A/D2 ratio). Although it is not clear if it is as effective as olanzapine and risperidone in the acute treatment of schizophrenia (McCue, Waheed, et al. 2006), it does not cause metabolic changes, and may even improve lipid profile, especially if the patient was previously on a weight gain-inducing agent (Lieberman, Stroup, et al. 2005). A major issue with using ziprasidone is the necessity of taking it with food, or it will not be well-absorbed. A 500 calorie meal is optimal with each of the twice daily doses (Miceli, Glue, et al. 2007). The optimal dose for ziprasidone is 80 mg twice daily: lower doses may not be different from placebo in schizophrenia (Citrome, Yang et al. 2009).

Ziprasidone has the potential to prolong QT more than other SGAs. Although a pre-treatment ECG is not required, those who are deemed, based on history or age, to be at higher cardiac risk would benefit from an ECG (and medical consultation if arrhythmias are present) before starting ziprasidone. It should be avoided if baseline QTc is greater or equal to 500 msec. Electrolyte disturbances such as hypomagnesemia and hypokalemia should be corrected. Other QT prolonging medications should not be used in combination with ziprasidone. Despite concerns regarding this effect, post-marketing studies (e.g., CATIE) (Lieberman, Stroup, et al. 2005) did not show any clinically significant QT prolongation with ziprasidone use.

Clinicians should be aware that all antipsychotics (with the possible exception of aripiprazole discussed below) could affect cardiac conduction, potentially delaying conduction enough to lead to fatal arrhythmias. There is an association between the use of antipsychotics (as well as tricyclic antidepressants) and sudden cardiac death (Ray, Chung, et al. 2009; Ray, Meredith, et al. 2004; Straus, Bleumink, et al. 2004). As discussed in the chapter on antidepressants, prolonged QTc is associated with torsades de pointes, a potentially fatal arrhythmia. The QT interval includes both the QRS interval as well as the ST segment. Whereas TCAs and some FGAs with tricyclic structure (e.g. chlorpromazine) lengthen the QRS interval by interfering with sodium channels and depolarization, most other antipsychotics, including SGAs, can affect potassium channels and the repolarization phase (Glassman and Bigger 2001). Both effects would be reflected in the QT interval. Although it is not clear if QT prolongation is always a reliable indicator of the risk of torsades, measuring this interval is the simplest way to estimate this risk (Shah 2005). Therefore, increases in the QTc interval above normal requires

ECG monitoring; a QTc of 500 msec or higher necessitates anti-psychotic discontinuation (Nielsen, Graff et al. 2011). In either case, any underlying hypokalemia or hypomagnesemia should be corrected. Investigation for any medical history of cardiac arrhythmias, cardiomyopathy, congenital prolonged QT, or syncope may also alert the clinician to those at higher risk of cardiac effects from the use of antipsychotics. In addition to ziprasidone, the FGAs thioridazine, **mesoridazine**, pimozide, and **droperidol** are among the antipsychotics with the highest propensity to prolong the QT interval (Fayek, Kingsbury, et al. 2001).

Aripiprazole, in contrast to other SGAs, is a high affinity partial agonist at the D2 receptor (Mamo, Graff, et al. 2007). It is proposed that aripiprazole decreases overall dopamine effect in dopamine rich environments (e.g., in mesolimbic pathways--thereby ameliorating psychosis), and increases dopamine effect in dopamine depleted environments (e.g., in mesocortical pathways to the prefrontal cortex--thereby improving negative symptoms such as social withdrawal) (Stahl 2008). At therapeutic doses it highly saturates the targeted dopamine receptors and shows very slow dissociation from the receptors upon discontinuation (Goff 2008; Grunder, Fellows, et al. 2008). It also shows moderate 5HT2A and 5HT2C antagonism. However, the theoretical ramifications of this pharmacodynamic profile (i.e., dopaminergic effect) do not seem to have been fully realized: efficacy appears to be only average (Osser, Roudsari et al. 2013). Aripiprazole's side effect profile is relatively mild, however. It is free from anticholinergic and significant antihistaminic effects. It has only small effects on QTc and cardiac function (El-Sayeh, Morganti, et al. 2006; Chung and Chua 2011) and only mild weight gain in chronic patients (Fava, Wisniewski et al. 2009). However, in adolescents and others receiving first time treatment with an antipsychotic, weight gain can be significant (e.g., 10 lbs. over 11 weeks) (Correll, Manu et al. 2009).

Aripiprazole carries a low risk of EPS, likely due to its partial agonism, rather than full antagonism, at D2 receptors, and it does not otherwise exhibit preferential extrastriatal D2 occupancy (Takahata, Ito et al. 2012). Although it is less likely to cause EPS in general, it has been observed in practice to cause akathisia more readily than other SGAs. This may occur early in treatment and is usually only mildly to moderately severe (Kane, Barnes et al. 2010). Akathisia may be more common if the patient was recently on a strong D2 antagonist such as an FGA or risperidone and consequently has an up-regulated or hypersensitive population of D2 receptors (Raja 2007).

Aripiprazole at 15 mg/day may be more efficacious than 30 mg/day in schizophrenia, although full response may take longer than with a comparable dose of haloperidol (Kane, Carson, et al. 2002). Higher doses (e.g. 30 mg/day) may be more useful in treatment-resistant schizophrenia (Kane, Meltzer, et al. 2007). Relapse rates may be somewhat higher with aripiprazole than with some other SGAs (Pigott, Carson, et al. 2003).

Clozapine, the first and in some respects the most impressive of the second generation antipsychotics, binds broadly to different dopamine receptors. It binds weakly to the D2 receptor, but shows relatively greater net antagonism at D4 dopamine receptors (Seeman 1992; Brunello, Masotto et al. 1995). It has moderate affinity for 5HT2A and 5HT2C receptors. It is often effective when other antipsychotics are not (Lewis, Barnes, et al. 2006), and appears to have superior antisuicidal effects in patients with schizophrenia or schizoaffective disorder (Meltzer, Alphs et al. 2003). However, because of an approximately 0.4-2% risk of agranulocytosis, most of which occurs between the first 6 weeks to 6 months of treatment (Honigfeld, Arellano et al. 1998; Meltzer 2012), it is reserved primarily for schizophrenia and schizoaffective patients who have failed to respond adequately to at least two other antipsychotics. However, it has FDA-approval for non-treatment-resistant schizophrenia patients with active suicidal ideation. Strict monitoring and blood draws initially weekly for the first 6 months, then biweekly for the next 6 months, and then every 4 weeks, are required to monitor white cell count. The clinician should consult the package insert and strictly follow the monitoring guidelines. Clozapine should not be combined with other medications (e.g., carbamazepine) that may also cause leukopenia.

Clozapine can also cause multiple other adverse effects, which include (but are not limited to) an increased risk of seizures, rare myocarditis, eosinophilia, anticholinergic and antihistaminic effects, orthostasis, weight gain and adverse metabolic effects (Lamberti, Olson, et al. 2006). Given the complicated nature of clozapine treatment, the clinician should refer to a more in depth discussion of this drug before use (Phansalkar and Osser 2009; Phansalkar and Osser 2009). Clozapine has multiple other potential side effects including severe constipation (because it is strongly anticholinergic), sedation, hypersalivation, tachycardia, and a low grade fever.

Among the SGAs, clozapine and olanzapine are the most likely (and aripiprazole, ziprasidone, asenapine, and lurasidone are the least likely) to cause adverse metabolic effects. These would include weight gain, hyperglycemia and diabetes (with or without weight gain) and hyperlipidemia (ADA 2004). A 2-3 kilogram weight gain within the first 3 weeks of treatment often predicts the risk of significant weight gain over the long term (Lipkovich, Citrome, et al. 2006). Decreased insulin secretion and increased triglycerides (i.e., the lipids most affected by SGAs) (Osser, Najarian, et al. 1999) can also be seen within 1-2 weeks of treatment (Chiu, Chen, et al. 2006), or even after a single dose of olanzapine (Hahn, Wolever et al. 2013).

Prior to starting olanzapine or clozapine, measurements of baseline weight, serum glucose, and lipid profile should be obtained. If the patient has pre-existing diabetes, other antispychotics should be considered. Once treatment is initiated, serum glucose and weight should be monitored and if glucose levels become elevated, a glucose tolerance test—which can predict up to 96% of patients who would develop diabetes—should be done (van Winkel, De Hert, et al. 2006). If metabolic problems do arise during treatment, switching to another antipsychotic should be considered. Treatment with the hypoglycemic medication metformin, especially if combined with lifestyle changes, may reduce antipsychotic-induced weight gain and metabolic effects (Baptista, Rangel, et al. 2007; Wu, Zhao, et al. 2008; Maayan, Vakhrusheva et al. 2010; Praharaj, Jana et al. 2011; Caemmerer, Correll et al. 2012; Correll, Sikich et al. 2013). Recent pharmacogenomic findings, such as an association between 5HT2C polymorphisms and antipsychotic induced weight gain (Sicard, Zai et al. 2010), may allow for better screening and personalization of treatment in the future.

Clozapine may cause orthostatic hypotension. Patients who are elderly, have cardiac histories, or who are taking antihypertensives are at higher risk for this side effect. Clozapine should be increased gradually after treatment is initiated (starting at 12.5 mg/day and increasing the dose by 25 mg daily as tolerated). Usually, patients adjust and become tolerant to the hypotensive effects of this medication. However, this tolerance may not last longer than 48 hours. If a patient discontinues clozapine therapy for more than 48 hours, treatment should be restarted with a 12.5 mg dose. After that, the dose may be more quickly raised to the previous dose as tolerated. It is important for the physician who may be admitting a psychiatric patient to the medical or surgical ward of the hospital to stop and think before continuing clozapine at its prior dose: recent compliance needs to be verified first.

Due to its many potential adverse effects, and the time required to monitor and manage these effects, clozapine is underutilized in the United States. Even though it is often effective when patients are treatment refractory to other antipsychotics, many clinicians choose to delay its appropriate use. When 2 or more adequate trials of antipsychotics have been ineffective in treating a patient's schizophrenia, it is often the case that psychiatrists opt for other, often unsuccessful, antipsychotic trials or combination antipsychotic treatments (for which there is very little supportive evidence), rather than offering clozapine (for which there is a significant evidence base). Consequently multiple failed trials and polypharmacy then may burden patients with increased adverse effects, and more importantly fail to adequately treat their psychotic illness. Clinicians should keep in mind that for many patients clozapine is likely to be more effective than other antipsychotics for treatment-resistant psychosis, reduce suicidality, have a low risk for tardive dyskinesia, improve quality of life, and decrease the risk of relapse (Meltzer 2012).

Newer Second Generation Antipsychotics

In the past few years, four new antipsychotics, namely **paliperidone**, **iloperidone**, **asenapine**, and **lurasidone** have been introduced in the United States. Their mechanism of action (i.e., dopamine receptor antagonism) is generally considered to be similar to those of the SGAs discussed above. Paliperidone, as noted below, behaves clinically in a similar manner to risperidone, its parent compound. The remaining three exhibit some variations in their effects on serotonin receptor subtypes, but it is not yet clear if any of these variations confer any added clinical benefit in either efficacy (in schizophrenia or schizoaffective disorder) or tolerability when compared to already available less costly antipsychotics. Differences do exist, however, among them in terms of side effect profiles. Relative to olanzapine and clozapine, iloperidone, asenapine, and lurasidone all appear to have relatively favorable metabolic risk profiles. However lurasidone and asenapine appear to have a significant risk of treatment emergent akathisia. None have been tested in first or early-onset schizophrenia patients nor have they been used in treatment-resistant patients, so their role remains unclear.

Paliperidone is the major active metabolite of risperidone (see above) and has similar efficacy and side effects. Because it is not metabolized by CYP2D6 and is mostly renally excreted, it is likely to have fewer drug-drug interactions (Wang, Han et al. 2012). However it may have a higher risk of QT prolongation (Suzuki, Fukui et al. 2012), more tachycardia, and possibly more EPS (although with similar propensity to increase prolactin) than risperidone (Nussbaum and Stroup 2012). It is significantly more expensive than its now generically available parent compound.

Iloperidone (not a metabolite or analogue of paliperidone or risperidone) is a D2 and 5HT2A receptor antagonist. It also has a high affinity for D3 and noradrenergic alpha-1 receptors, and moderate affinity for D4, 5HT6 and 5HT7 receptors. Alpha-1 blockade results in a significant propensity to cause orthostasis, thereby requiring slow dose titration. It is thought to carry a very low risk of causing EPS or akathisia, and has little effect on prolactin levels. Moderate weight gain (more than risperidone but without significant change in glucose or lipids) and mild sedation can occur. QT prolongation may be higher than with some other antipsychotics (Citrome 2010; Weiden 2012).

Asenapine, another D2 and 5HT2 antagonist, is also a partial agonist at the 5HT1A receptor. It also shows high affinity and antagonism for a broad range of other 5HT receptors and dopamine receptors, the clinical relevance of which is unclear. Asenapine is associated with low metabolic risks, low risk of prolactin elevation, and mild EPS risk; however dose dependent akathisia may occur. It is the first sublingually administered antipsychotic and the twice-daily doses must be held under the tongue for 10 minutes; if swallowed too soon absorption will be poor. Usage is associated with oral numbing which may also affect compliance (Potkin 2011; Stoner and Pace 2012; Tarazi and Stahl 2012). Severe and potentially lethal allergic reactions may occur with asenapine, even after the first dose (FDA 2011).

Lurasidone is a potent D2 and 5HT2A antagonist. It also acts as a potent 5HT7 antagonist and a 5HT1A agonist, and it is not yet clear how these receptor effects might influence clinical efficacy (although based on animal studies, effects on cognition, depression, and anxiety have been proposed) (Ishibashi, Horisawa et al. 2010; Risbood, Lee et al. 2012). It is associated with minimal weight gain and appears to have a low risk of metabolic side effects; and it may have no significant effect on QT prolongation (Kantrowitz and Citrome 2012; Risbood, Lee et al. 2012). Prolactin elevation may occur and a dose dependent increase in parkinsonism, akathisia and somnolence may be observed (McIntyre, Cha et al. 2012; Risbood, Lee et al. 2012). It should be taken once a day with a 350 calorie meal.

Time to Response

Antipsychotics, whether first or second generation, do not have full immediate antipsychotic effect. Sedation, which can be a non-specific side effect of most but not all antipsychotics, may immediately decrease assaultiveness and agitation should these be present. Historically, when antipsychotics were first introduced, significant improvement was observed over many months. A therapeutic sequence of initially diminished assaultiveness and increased cooperation (within the first week), followed by gradual socialization while psychosis persisted (within 4-6 weeks), followed sometimes by the complete elimination of thought disorder over many months, was observed when FGAs were first used (Lehman 1964).

Today, managed care organizations often choose to presume that significant improvement, e.g. improvement that would allow discharge from the hospital, could be expected in as soon as a week. This is likely to be too optimistic. It may be reasonable to expect that a quarter of treated first-episode schizophrenia patients could show a modest 20% or greater improvement in rating scales within the first week, however a third of the patients may require 4-8 weeks for similar response (Emsley, Rabinowitz et al. 2006). However, the lack of any response within the first 2 weeks of treatment, a period within which some clear response is often noted (Jager, Riedel et al. 2010), predicts poor response within 3 months. No response in 2 weeks may therefore suggest the need for change in dose or type of antipsychotic (Leucht, Busch et al. 2007). Clinicians should keep in mind however that antipsychotics vary in their speed of response (e.g., quicker response may be seen with risperidone) (Osser and Sigadel 2001). Temporary sedation with adjunctive benzodiazapines may also be a reasonably safe way to speed progress to dischargeability (Osser, Roudsari et al. 2013). Treatment-resistant patients may require a longer time to respond.

Long-Acting Injectable Antipsychotics

In the United States, six antipsychotics are available for long-acting (i.e., depot) intramuscular administration: **haloperidol decanoate, fluphenazine decanoate, long-acting injectable risperidone, olanzapine long-acting injection, paliperidone long-acting injectable, and aripiprazole long-acting injectable.** These long-acting formulations are options for patients who are frequently non-adherent to the oral medication (Olfson, Marcus, et al. 2007). A trial of the antipsychotic in oral form is generally prescribed first to assess patients' response to, and tolerance of, the selected agent. Depending on which agent is used, injections would then be given every 2 or 4 weeks. For example, every four-week injections of haloperidol decanoate or biweekly injections of long-acting fluphenazine or risperidone are then continued while the oral agent is gradually tapered. Two to six weeks of the selected antipsychotic may be necessary while waiting for the depot to achieve steady state before oral medications should be completely withdrawn (Osser and Sigadel 2001). Unfortunately, patients who adhere poorly to oral medications in real-world community settings where follow-up services may be suboptimal are generally non-adherent to depot antipsychotics as well (Olfson, Marcus, et al. 2007). Although some studies suggest that depot antipsychotics can reduce relapse, the findings appear to be limited by many of these studies' methodological problems (Leucht, Heres et al. 2011; Osser, Roudsari et al. 2013). Long-acting formulations seem to work best in research subjects and in other populations of relatively cooperative and less firmly non-adherent patients who have good support in the community. On the other hand, once steady state is achieved, depots do have the advantage that if the patient discontinues treatment, the antipsychotic effect can continue for up to several months after the last received dose; this gives some time for other interventions to be employed.

Antipsychotics for Acute Behavioral Control

Both SGAs and FGAs are used in psychiatric practice to treat behavioral agitation. In acutely psychotic and/or manic patients, FGAs, such as oral or intramuscular haloperidol (invariably combined with lorazcpam and/or benztropine to decrease the risk of acute dystonias), remain the mainstay of treatment (Ansari, Osser, et al. 2009; Osser, Roudsari et al. 2013). Intramuscular fluphenazine can also be considered in place of haloperidol if the patient has a haloperidol allergy. Newer antipsychotics, such as olanzapine, ziprasidone, and aripiprazole are also available in short-acting intramuscular form but they are expensive and seem to have no advantage in effectiveness or side effects when compared with the combination therapy noted above (Satterthwaite, Wolf, et al. 2008), and in a recent controlled study were inferior in one or the other of these respects (Mantovani, Labate et al. 2013). When considering antipsychotics for behavioral agitation, clinicians should be advised not to use (1) intramuscular droperidol due to high risk of QT prolongation, (2) intramuscular chlorpromazine due to risk of severe hypotension and no greater effectiveness vs. haloperidol (Ahmed, Jones et al. 2010), (3) intramuscular ziprasidone if the patient is taking other medications that can also prolong QT including oral ziprasidone, or (4) intramuscular olanzapine in combination with lorazepam or other benzodiazepines due to the risk of hypotension (Zacher and Roche-Desilets 2005).

The use of antipsychotics for the treatment of behavioral agitation in elderly patients with dementia is problematic both in terms of effectiveness and tolerability.

First, in terms of effect, they do not appear to provide more than minimal benefit in targeting symptoms of agitation (Cheung and Stapelberg 2011), and SGAs may not be different from placebo in this regard (Yury and Fisher 2007). The NIMH-sponsored CATIE-AD study, which studied the effectiveness of olanzapine, quetiapine and risperidone in the treatment of symptoms of psychosis, aggression and agitation in patients with Alzheimer's disease, also found that even when these symptoms did improve with treatment, the antipsychotic did not improve overall functioning (Sultzer, Davis, et al. 2008). Furthermore, any improvement in specific symptoms was offset by adverse effects and led to overall discontinuation rates (when both efficacy and tolerability were considered) that were no different from placebo (Schneider, Tariot, et al. 2006). Secondly, antipsychotics have been found to be associated with an increased risk of stroke in patients with dementia and an overall increased risk of adverse medical events and death in this population (Gill, Rochon, et al. 2005; Herrmann and Lanctot 2005; Rochon, Normand, et al. 2008; Schneider, Dagerman, et al. 2005). Both FGAs and SGAs appear to increase the risk of death in patients with dementia (Schneeweiss, Setoguchi, et al. 2007; Wang, Schneeweiss, et al. 2005). Nevertheless, it should be noted that despite all these safety concerns, if immediate relief from dangerous behavior is required (as in periods of hospitalization), antipsychotics may still need to be considered in behaviorally dysregulated patients with dementia. Non-psychopharmacological and non-antipsychotic interventions however should also be concurrently considered.

High-potency FGAs are also often used in the treatment of delirium in hospitalized patients (Lonergan, Britton, et al. 2007). SGAs such as olanzapine, risperidone, and quetiapine may also be efficacious (Tahir, Eeles et al. 2010; Grover, Mattoo et al. 2011). Still, there is little reason to choose more costly SGAs over haloperidol for delirium. Clinicians should be aware that although antipsychotics may treat the secondary manifestations of delirium, such as behavioral agitation and/or hallucinations, they do not treat the underlying condition. Delirium is a medical condition that should be treated by addressing the underlying medical cause.

Antipsychotics for Non-Psychotic Disorders

SGAs have been studied for use in non-psychotic disorders and some have Food and Drug Administration (FDA) indications for their use in these disorders. However, given issues related to the long-term risks associated with antipsychotics, it is important to consider less problematic alternatives prior to considering the use of antipsychotics in most non-psychotic disorders. Depending on the diagnosis, they should generally be considered for short-term use only and should be tapered off when no longer needed. They do have an important role in the treatment of bipolar disorder that is discussed below and in the chapter on mood stabilizers.

SGAs, particularly quetiapine, may help with symptomatic relief of anxiety symptoms, and have been studied for generalized anxiety disorder (Bandelow, Chouinard et al. 2010; Depping,

Komossa et al. 2010; Katzman, Brawman-Mintzer et al. 2011; Khan, Joyce et al. 2011). None of the SGAs however have been approved by the FDA for this indication due to their severe side effects compared to other effective agents.

Several SGAs have been studied for augmentation of antidepressants in treatment-resistant unipolar depression (Spielmans, Berman et al. 2013). Aripiprazole at lower than usual doses (average 10 mg per day) may be efficacious when added to an antidepressant and tolerable in the short run (Berman, Marcus et al. 2007; Khan 2008; Marcus, McQuade et al. 2008; Nelson, Thase et al. 2012). Olanzapine, quetiapine (extended release), and risperidone may also reduce depressive symptoms when added to an antidepressant (Spielmans, Berman et al. 2013). In general, about 9 patients must be treated with SGA augmentation before one patient's improvement is noted that would not have occurred on placebo. However, the risk of serious side effects (e.g., weight gain) is much higher. Older augmentation strategies such as the addition of a second antidepressant, buspirone, lithium or thyroid hormone to a partially effective antidepressant should be considered prior to considering SGA augmentation, despite the intense marketing associated with the SGAs at this time.

Antipsychotics are frequently used in the treatment of patients with bipolar disorder. Traditionally, FGAs have been used for their sedative effects on acutely agitated manic patients. SGAs have been found effective and are FDA approved for the acute treatment of mania (Perlis, Welge et al. 2006). They are also frequently used in conjunction with a mood stabilizer. Both work equally well as monotherapy and it is not clear if they bring about a quicker anti-manic response when used together: it usually takes 3-4 weeks for improvement and more time for remission in mania. Of note however, in the depressive phase of bipolar disorder, not all SGAs are equally efficacious. Quetiapine is particularly effective in bipolar depression (and along with lithium) may be considered one of the first-line treatments for this condition (Ansari and Osser 2010). Olanzapine (in combination with fluoxetine) has also been found to have some efficacy in treating bipolar depression. However, poorer longer-term tolerability of the olanzapine component limits its use. Most recently, lurasidone was found to be efficacious and approved for acute bipolar depression (Loebel, Cucchiaro et al. 2014), though it has not yet been studied in mania. Several SGAs are also FDA approved for adjunctive use with lithium or valproate for acute and maintenance treatment. However given the long-term risk of SGAs, they should not be used for maintenance unless monotherapy with mood stabilizers such as lithium is ineffective or not tolerated.

In summary, antipsychotics are being considered and used in a wide variety of mood and anxiety disorders as augmentations when antidepressants produce unsatisfactory results, and sometimes they are used as primary treatments for these disorders. Recent data indicating that SGAs and FGAs are associated with double to triple the rate of death from sudden cardiac arrest (presumably from electrophysiological effects related to QT prolongation) suggest that these agents should not be first-line treatments in these clinical situations (Ray, Chung, et al. 2009). However, antipsychotics are powerful and important options in the treatment of schizophrenia and severe bipolar disorders and these new cardiac concerns should not deter clinicians for prescribing them appropriately for these patients. Obtaining a baseline ECG, and if abnormal obtaining another after dosage has been optimized, is a prudent risk-management approach given these new data.

Further Notes on the Clinical Use of Antipsychotics

Comparative Studies and Meta-analyses: All antipsychotics are indicated for the treatment of schizophrenia and are considered reasonably safe and effective for this debilitating disorder. However, there has been much debate about whether there are efficacy differences among these medications, or whether the side effect differences, which are considerable, should be the primary basis for selecting a medication for a particular patient. A meta-analysis of 78 head-to-head comparisons in the literature through 2007 concluded that the efficacy differences are small, but there was some superiority to olanzapine and risperidone, when compared with aripiprazole, quetiapine, and ziprasidone (Leucht, Komossa et al. 2009). A problem with this meta-analysis, however, was that almost all of the studies were industry-sponsored. Such studies invariably find outcomes in favor of the sponsor's product, and olanzapine and risperidone have sponsored the largest number of studies.

Another meta-analysis focused on 150 studies that directly compared FGAs with SGAs.(Leucht, Corves, et al. 2009) The authors found that clozapine was clearly superior to the others especially for positive symptoms of hallucinations and delusions. Olanzapine and risperidone were superior to the rest, but with a small effect size. After that, there were no differences in efficacy. The side effect profiles differed markedly, with no pattern to the differences. The authors recommended abandoning the terms "FGA" and "SGA" as irrelevant to efficacy or side effects.

CATIE: Many clinicians put more reliance on the few comparison studies that were independently funded, such as the CATIE (Clinical Antipsychotics Trials of Intervention Effectiveness) study (Lieberman, Stroup, et al. 2005), funded by the U.S. National Institute of Mental Health. This study prospectively compared the FGA perphenazine, with SGAs (clozapine, olanzapine, risperidone, quetiapine, ziprasidone) and found generally no differences in effectiveness except that clozapine was superior. There were no differences in the ability to improve impaired cognition, despite prior claims for SGA superiority from studies sponsored by the SGA pharmaceutical firms (Keefe, Bilder, et al. 2007). None worked well for this, and there was thus no evidence of a 'neuroprotective effect' of SGAs.

Some experts have interpreted CATIE as showing olanzapine to be superior to the other non-clozapine antipsychotics, but this seems likely to be due to peculiar results with the cohort of patients who were on olanzapine prior to entering the CATIE study. These patients (22% of the sample) were randomly assigned to either continue on olanzapine or be switched to one of the other options in CATIE (perphenazine, risperidone, quetiapine, or ziprasidone). The patients who were assigned to remain on olanzapine did better than those who were abruptly switched to any of the other options (Essock, Covell, et al. 2006). By contrast, the patients who entered the study on risperidone (the second largest group with 19%) showed no advantage to staying on risperidone compared to switching to another agent. Notably, there was no advantage to switching to olanzapine. Hence, the superiority of olanzapine seen in CATIE may be due to the study having a large sample of patients who had been previously stabilized on olanzapine and who clearly responded only to olanzapine or who may have been more prone to a withdrawal-induced exacerbation when taken off of olanzapine. Since olanzapine has a very unfavorable side effect profile with its tendency to promote weight gain, insulin resistance, and the metabolic syndrome, this would appear to make it undesirable as a first-line choice even if it does have slightly superior efficacy.

Other findings from CATIE could be summarized as follows: (1) The FGA perphenazine was generally at least as effective as the SGAs quetiapine, risperidone and ziprasidone, and was the most cost-effective; however more patients on perphenazine had EPS; (2) those who discontinued the FGA perphenazine subsequently did better on olanzapine or quetiapine rather than on risperidone, the SGA with the strongest D2 affinity; (3) olanzapine and risperidone were generally more effective than quetiapine and ziprasidone (although see caveats above for olanzapine); (4) in terms of side effects, patients on olanzapine had the most metabolic side effects, risperidone was associated with hyperprolactinemia, and ziprasidone did not show any clinically relevant QT prolongation; (5) clozapine worked best in treatment-resistant patients. These findings suggest that antipsychotics are not equally effective and tolerability profiles are variable. As always, treatment of patients with schizophrenia should be customized to meet each patient's individual needs and profiles (Keefe, Bilder et al. 2007; Swartz, Stroup et al. 2008; Lieberman and Stroup 2011).

Notes on the Implications of the New Diagnostic and Statistical Manual of Mental Disorders, 5th Edition (DSM-5) Criteria for Psychotic Disorders

DSM-5 was released in 2013 (APA 2013). In DSM-IV the criteria for schizoaffective disorder were difficult to apply and produced much inter-rater unreliability. The new DSM-5 criteria correct this and expand the diagnosis of schizophrenia by allowing diagnosed patients to meet full criteria for a mood syndrome (mania or depression) during up to 49% of the total duration of their illness course to date. Before, mood episodes could only be "brief" relative to the total duration of the illness: in an example provided in DSM-IV brief was defined as 2.5% of the time. The consequences of this change in DSM-5 are that fewer psychotic patients will be diagnosed with schizoaffective disorder and more will be diagnosed with schizophrenia. This suggests that fewer psychotic patients with mood symptoms should receive prescriptions for antidepressants and mood stabilizers along with their antipsychotic. These medications for mood symptoms have little evidence of efficacy targeting those symptoms in schizophrenia.

Future Trends

Despite the recent introduction of multiple new antipsychotics, the pharmacological treatment of schizophrenia has changed very little and continues to rely on agents that primarily exert their therapeutic effects through dopamine antagonism. Alternately however, the observation that antagonists (e.g., ketamine, dextromethorphan, phencyclidine) at the N-methyl-D-aspartate (NMDA) receptor (a specific type of glutamate receptor) can cause psychosis, has increased interest in the glutamatergic system (Nestler, Hyman, et al. 2009; de Bartolomeis, Sarappa et al. 2012). Glutamate and glycine bind to these receptors and activate them. Oral glycine and glycine agonists, such as D-cycloserine and D-serine, have been studied and have shown mixed results in animal and human studies of schizophrenia. Of note, clozapine, which appears to be a particularly effective antipsychotic, has also been shown to interact with glutamate receptors (Schwieler, Linderholm et al. 2008). Still, NMDA agonists have not yet been consistently shown to have clinically significant effects in humans (de Bartolomeis, Sarappa et al. 2012). Another important and promising new development is the use of sodium nitroprusside in patients with schizophrenia (Hallak, Maia-de-Oliveira et al. 2013). In this small but placebo-controlled study, subjects showed significant improvements after a 4 hour infusion of nitroprusside when compared to placebo, and these improvements lasted up to 4 weeks. The mechanism of action is thought to involve the interaction between glutamate and nitic oxide; sodium nitroprusside enhances nitric oxide production in the brain. Lastly, anti-inflammatory drugs, added to antipsychotics, have also been studied and may show some promise in decreasing the severity of psychotic symptoms in schizophrenic patients, but further study is needed in this regard (Laan, Grobbee et al. 2010; Sommer, de Witte et al. 2012; Sommer, van Westrhenen et al. 2014).

Table of Antipsychotics

Table 3 summarizes the characteristics of commonly used antipsychotics (Ansari and Osser 2009; WHO 2011; PDR 2014).

TABLE 3. COMMONLY USED ANTIPSYCHOTICS

MEDICATION*	DOSING**	COMMENTS/ *FDA Indication*
Chlorpromazine (FGA) (Thorazine®)	For oral: Start: 25-50 mg po qhs then increase as tolerated to 300 mg po qhs or in divided doses. Potency: 100 mg po equals haloperidol 2 mg po.	Tricyclic structure therefore with TCA side effects, plus EPS; now rarely used as primary antipsychotic; avoid IM given risk of severe orthostasis. On WHO Essential Medicines List for psychotic disorders. *Psychotic disorders/Other indications (see package insert)*
Thioridazine (FGA) (Mellaril®)	Start: 25 mg po q day/bid/tid for agitation in a variety of anxiety, mood, personality disorders; for schizophrenia increase the same as chlorpromazine. Potency: 80-100 mg po equals haloperidol 2 mg po.	Was once the most frequently prescribed antipsychotic; now should avoid use due to the highest risk of QTc prolongation of all FGAs and SGAs; doses over 800 mg/day may cause pigmentary retinopathy; CYP2D6 substrate, avoid combining with CYP2D6 inhibitors or any SSRI or propranolol. *Schizophrenia in patients not responsive to or intolerant to other antipsychotics*
Perphenazine (FGA) (Trilafon®)	Start: 4 mg po bid then increase by 4-8 mg every 2 days; 20-24 mg/day in divided doses may be sufficient, 40 mg/day in treatment resistant patients, maximum dose 64 mg/day. Potency: 8-10 mg po equals haloperidol 2mg po.	Effective in recent studies in comparison with SGAs; good choice for a first-line FGA. CYP2D6 substrate. *Schizophrenia*
Pimozide (FGA)	Start: 0.5 mg po q day,	Avoid use; historically used

(Orap®)	increase very gradually if needed and maintain low doses (less than stated maximum of 10 mg/day). Potency: 1 mg po equals haloperidol 2 mg po.	for delusional parasitosis but no reason to believe better for this than others; high risk of QTc prolongation; CYP3A4, CYP1A2, CYP2D6 substrate. *Suppression of refractory tics secondary to Tourette's Syndrome who failed to respond to standard therapy*
Fluphenazine (FGA) (Prolixin®)	For oral: Start: 0.5-2 mg po bid and increase as tolerated and necessary, usual daily dose is 5-10 mg/day. PO max is 40 mg/day IM max is 20 mg/day Oral dose is equipotent with haloperidol	Available in short-acting IM for behavioral control and long-acting injectable depot preparation for maintenance treatment of poorly adherent patients given every 2 weeks (see package insert); On WHO Essential Medicines List for psychotic disorders. *Psychotic disorders*
Haloperidol (FGA) (Haldol®)	For oral: Start: 0.5-2 mg po q day or bid and increase as tolerated and necessary, lower doses for elderly delirious patients and higher doses in patients with schizophrenia, 4-10 mg/day may be sufficient in schizophrenia	Most widely used FGA; also used for secondary symptoms of delirium and behavioral control; available in short-acting IM form for behavioral control and long-acting injectable depot form for maintenance treatment given every 4 weeks (see package insert); CYP2D6, CYP3A4 substrate. On WHO Essential Medicines List for psychotic disorders. *Schizophrenia/other indications (see package insert)*
Risperidone (SGA) (Risperdal®, Risperdal M-Tab®, Risperdal Consta®)	For oral risperidone, Risperdal, Risperdal M-Tab: Start: 0.5-1 mg po bid and increase gradually every	Fairly well-tolerated SGA, usually no significant EPS under 4 mg/day, and medium to low risk of metabolic changes in adults; orthostasis

	1-2 days to target of 4 mg/day, if no response in 1-2 weeks then increase to 6 mg/day.	may be a problem initially; hyperprolactinemia is common; may have more rapid action than other SGAs; available in long-acting injectable depot form for maintenance treatment given every 2 weeks (see package insert); CYP2D6 substrate. *Schizophrenia/Psychotic disorders/Acute mania or mixed episodes/Irritability from autism (see package insert)*
Olanzapine (SGA) (Zyprexa®, Zydis®, Zyprexa IntraMuscular®, Zyprexa Relprevv®, Symbyax®—olanzapine, fluoxetine combination)	For oral olanzapine, Zyprexa, Zydis: Start: 15 mg/day for most rapid effect in male smokers for schizophrenia; 10 mg in women smokers; 5 mg in non-smoking women. May increase by 5 mg/day until 15-20 mg/day, (package insert max is 20 mg/day for oral, and 30 mg/day for short acting injectable), otherwise see package insert for short-acting intramuscular use.	Along with clozapine the highest risk of weight gain and metabolic syndrome among SGAs; CYP1A2, CYP2D6 substrate. For long acting injection steady state is achieved after 3 months; "post-injection delirium sedation syndrome" may occur from inadvertent IV administration, within 5 hours of injection. See package insert for q 2-4 week long-acting injectable. *Schizophrenia/Acute treatment of mania or mixed episodes/Bipolar Maintenance/ As adjunct to lithium or valproate for treatment of manic or mixed episodes/ For acute agitation associated with schizophrenia or mania/ In combination with fluoxetine for treatment-resistant depression or bipolar depression*
Quetiapine (SGA)	For non-XR: Start: 25-50	Efficacious in bipolar

(Seroquel®, Seroquel XR®)	mg po bid and double daily until 100 mg bid then increase by 200 mg/day as tolerated depending on sedation and orthostasis to 600-800 mg/day in schizophrenia or mania. Usual dose for acute bipolar depression is 300 mg per day. XR is once-daily version: 200 mg po qhs on day one, 400 mg po qhs on day 2, 600 mg po qhs on day 3. Max dose is 800 mg/day.	depression; used frequently off-label as anti-anxiety agent in substance abusers, and in personality disordered; CYP3A4, and CYP2D6 substrate. *Schizophrenia/Acute mania, alone or as adjunct to lithium or valproate/Bipolar I/II depression/Maintenance treatment of bipolar I disorder as adjunct to lithium or divalproex/ For treatment-resistant depression as adjunct to an antidepressant (for XR formulation)*
Ziprasidone (SGA) (Geodon®, Geodon for Injection®)	For oral: Start: 20-40 mg po bid and increase dose every 1-2 days to 80 mg po bid (need to take with 500 kcal of food for adequate absorption—see text) Max is 80 mg bid.	SGA with low risk of weight gain and metabolic side effects; SGA with highest risk of QTc prolongation; available in short-acting IM form for behavioral control (see package insert); CYP3A4, CYP1A2 substrate. *Schizophrenia/Acute mania or mixed episodes/Monotherapy or as adjunct to lithium or valproate for maintenance for bipolar I/Acute agitation in schizophrenia*
Aripiprazole (SGA) (Abilify®, Abilify Discmelt®, Abilify Injection®, Abilify Maintena®)	For oral: in schizophrenia and mania, start and stay at 15 mg po q am as tolerated, maximum is 30 mg/day but 15 mg/day may be more effective in acute schizophrenia; in mania 15 mg and 30 mg appear equally effective. For Maintena: give 400 mg IM every 4 weeks, may decrease to 300 mg	SGA with low risk of cardiac and metabolic effects; however akathisia is common; very long half-life; available in short-acting IM form for behavioral control; See package insert for short-acting and long-acting injectable forms. CYP2D6 and CYP3A4 substrate.

	for tolerability, continue oral for 2 weeks.	*Schizophrenia/Acute treatment of mixed/manic episodes/ Maintenance treatment as monotherapy or adjunct to lithium or valproate for Bipolar I/ Adjunctive therapy to antidepressants for acute treatment of MDD/Irritability associated with autistic disorder in ages 6-17. For injection: Agitation associated with schizophrenia or bipolar disorder.*
Clozapine (SGA) (Clozaril®, FazaClo®)	Start: 12.5 mg po once or twice daily then increase by 25 mg/day in divided doses as tolerated to 200-400 mg/day and check for response (check serum level if no response— therapeutic serum level of clozapine is over 350 ng/mL, some studies suggest over 450 ng/mL), need to restart at 12.5 mg/day if discontinued 48 hours or more	Risk of agranulocytosis; need WBC/ANC count and ECG before treatment; needs ongoing WBC monitoring— see package insert for WBC monitoring guidelines; multiple other risks; along with lithium may be one of only two drugs with antisuicidal effects; use caution when using with benzodiazepines; do not combine with carbamazepine; CYP1A2, CYP2D6, CYP3A4 substrate. *Treatment resistant severe schizophrenia/Reduction of recurrent suicidal behavior in chronically at risk patients with schizophrenia or schizoaffective disorder* (do not have to be treatment resistant for this latter indication)
NEWER ANTIPSYCHOTICS:		
Paliperidone (SGA) (Invega®) (Invega Sustenna®)	For oral: Start: 6 mg po daily, increase by 3 mg/day every 3-5 days if needed. Most	Major metabolite of risperidone. Available only in extended release capsules; gradual release may have less

	patients will require up to 12 mg po daily; max is 12 mg/day.	effect on acute agitation and anxiety; significant risk of EPS with upper end of dosing, higher QT prolongations than risperidone. For long-acting IM: See package insert, starting with 2 IM injections one week apart then every 4 weeks. Primarily excreted by kidneys so decreased drug-drug interactions. *Schizophrenia/Schizoaffective Disorder*
Iloperidone (SGA) (Fanapt®)	Start: 1 mg po bid, increase by 1-2 mg per day increments, target dose is 6-12 mg bid; max is 12 mg bid. Titrate slowly over first 7 days to avoid postural hypotension	Moderate weight gain, otherwise low metabolic risks, low risks of EPS or akathisia, risk of QT prolongation. CYP3A4 and CYP2D6 substrate *Schizophrenia*
Asenapine (SGA) (Saphris®)	Sublingual only, not to eat or drink for 10 minutes after each dose. If swallowed only 5% bioavailability because of liver metabolism to inactive compounds. Associated with oral numbing. Start: 5 mg SL bid for schizophrenia; 10 mg bid for mania. Max is 10 mg bid.	Low metabolic risks, mild EPS. Risk of dose-dependent akathisia. FDA warning about severe allergic reactions even after first dose. Extensively metabolized by liver. CYP1A2 substrate *Schizophrenia, Bipolar I disorder, acute mixed or manic episode, monotherapy or as adjunct to lithium or valproate.*
Lurasidone (SGA) (Latuda®)	Start: 40 mg po daily, maximum of 80 mg daily.	Low metabolic risk, low QT prolongation risk. Risk of

Should be taken with (350 calories) food. Although package insert max is 160 mg/day, doses higher than 60-80 mg/day show no added benefit.	dose-dependent akathisia. CYP3A4 substrate, and is itself a weak CYP3A4 inhibitor
	Schizophrenia

*Generic and U.S. brand name(s). ** Doses are provided for educational purposes only; see package insert for dosing and other information before prescribing medications. Dosing should be adjusted downward, ('start low, go slow' strategy) for the elderly and/or the medically compromised. Abbreviations: ANC-Absolute Neutrophil Count; bid-(bis in die) twice a day; CYP-Cytochrome P450 enzyme; ECG-Electrocardiogram; EPS-Extra-pyramidal Symptoms; FGA-First Generation Antipsychotics; IM-intramuscular; MDD-Major Depressive Disorder; mg-milligram; ng/mL-nanogram per milliliter; po-(per os) orally; q-(quaque) every; qhs-(quaque hora somni) at bedtime; SGA-Second Generation Antipsychotics; SL-sublingual; TCA-Tricyclic Antidepressants; WBC-White Blood Cell; WHO-World Health Organization.

MOOD STABILIZERS

What is a mood stabilizer? Although there is no generally accepted definition, a mood stabilizer can be defined as a medication that can treat either phase of bipolar disorder while not inducing or worsening the other phase. More conservatively, however, a mood stabilizer can be defined as an agent that has been shown to both treat *and prevent* both manic and depressive episodes. By this "two by two" definition only lithium qualifies as a true mood stabilizer (Bauer and Mitchner 2004).

Lithium (as a salt) has been used as a homeopathic treatment for gout and other disorders since the 1800's. Its calming effect on animals, and subsequently on manic patients, was first described in the 1940s (Cade 1949). In the brain, lithium inhibits inositol phosphatases that dephosphorylate inositol phosphates that are generated by the stimulation of G proteins in neuronal membranes activated by a neurotransmitter. This inhibition interferes with inositol regeneration and leads to its depletion in neurons, ultimately leading to decreased neuronal activity (Berridge, Downes et al. 1989; Harwood 2005; Serretti, Drago et al. 2009). Lithium also inhibits protein kinases, glycogen synthase kinase-3beta, and adenylyl cyclase (Bachmann, Schloesser, et al. 2005; Lenox and Hahn 2000), and may increase the uptake of the excitatory neurotransmitter glutamate thereby reducing glutamate activity at the neuronal synapse (Shaldubina, Agam, et al. 2001). Lithium also appears to have neuroprotective properties and may promote neurogenesis (Chuang 2005; Chen and Manji 2006; Bearden, Thompson, et al. 2007; Nunes, Forlenza, et al. 2007; Fornai, Longone, et al. 2008; Moore, Cortese et al. 2009; Lyoo, Dager et al. 2010; Hajek, Bauer et al. 2012; Hajek, Kopecek et al. 2012). Lithium is effective in both manic and depressive episodes associated with bipolar disorder, as well as for long-term maintenance. It is also the only mood stabilizer with anti-suicidal effect (Baldessarini, Tondo et al. 1999; Cipriani, Pretty et al. 2005; Cipriani, Hawton et al. 2013). This effect is distinct from its mood stabilizing properties (Ahrens and Muller-Oerlinghausen 2001). Lithium also works particularly well in patients who have a strong family history of bipolar disorder (Alda 1999).

A target therapeutic serum level of 0.6-0.75 mEq/L is recommended for the treatment of bipolar depression and prophylaxis against depressive relapses (Kleindienst, Severus, et al. 2007; Kleindienst, Severus, et al. 2005; Severus, Kleindienst, et al. 2008). Serum levels of 0.75-1.2 mEQ/L may be more effective for the treatment of mania and for treatment-resistant depression. Serum levels higher than 1.2 mEq/L are associated with significant lithium toxicity. ECG changes, namely QTc prolongation, may also occur more readily with serum levels greater than 1.2 mEq/L (Hsu, Liu et al. 2005).

Lithium side effects usually increase with higher serum doses but can occur at any dose. These may include nausea, vomiting, diarrhea, tremor, thirst, polyuria, acne, and a benign leukocytosis. Metabolic and hormonal side effects may include weight gain, nephrogenic diabetes insipidus, hyperparathyroidism and hypothyroidism (Livingstone and Rampes 2006). Over the long run, lithium can cause hypothyroidism in up to 20% of patients (Johnston and Eagles 1999) (which can be treated with thyroid hormone replacement), and worsening renal function in 20% of patients (Lepkifker, Sverdlik, et al. 2004) (which usually necessitates lithium discontinuation). Serious renal impairment is much less common, occurring in a placebo-corrected rate of about 0.3% (Bendz, Schon et al. 2010). Kidney functions must be monitored regularly (Jefferson 2010). Because of the many complexities of lithium use, access to relevant online or textbook references is recommended.

Clinicians should be aware that the anti-manic effects of lithium (and putative mood stabilizers, such as valproate and carbamazepine, discussed below) might not be achieved until 7-10 days after a therapeutic dose has been established. In the interim, sedative medications such as antipsychotics and benzodiazepines may be needed when the patient is acutely manic. Once the patient is stabilized, these adjunctive medications can often be tapered and lithium continued as monotherapy.

Valproate (along with carbamazepine and lamotrigine discussed below) is an anticonvulsant with putative mood stabilizing properties. It is postulated that it exerts its effect via enhancement of GABA transmission (Johannessen 2000). Despite decades of clinical experience with lithium, valproate has become the most widely used mood stabilizer in the United States. This is primarily due to its ease of use and effective marketing by its manufacturer. Some small studies show efficacy in the treatment of bipolar depression, but most emphasis has been on use in manic and mixed episodes (Bowden, Brugger, et al. 1994; Freeman, Clothier, et al. 1992). However, recent studies in mania have failed to show differences from placebo (Wagner, Redden et al. 2009;

Hirschfeld, Bowden et al. 2010), and overall valproate seems less effective than other agents for mania (Cipriani, Barbui et al. 2011). Although serum levels of 50-125 mcg/mL are generally considered to be within the therapeutic range (a range based on anticonvulsant usage), the best results in acute mania may occur with levels of greater than 90 mcg/mL (Allen, Hirschfeld, et al. 2006). Side effects in adults may include usually benign and transient liver enzyme elevations (severe hepatotoxicity and pancreatitis may be more common in the very young), nausea and diarrhea, hyperammonemia, alopecia, weight gain, and possible thrombocytopenia and platelet dysfunction. Because of the latter, bleeding time should be measured prior to surgery even if the platelet count is normal (De Berardis, Campanella, et al. 2003; Gerstner, Teich, et al. 2006). Valproate is highly protein-bound: concurrent use with warfarin can displace and increase the free fraction of warfarin and increase prothrombin time.

The use of valproate is problematic in women of child-bearing age. It is associated with a high risk of teratogenic effects (i.e., neural tube defects and decreased IQ scores) (Cohen 2007; Viguera, Koukopoulos, et al. 2007; Meador, Baker et al. 2009; PDR 2014). Because of this, a 2013 black box warning in the package insert recommends avoiding it in these women for all indications unless other reasonable options are not feasible. Valproate may also play a role in the development of polycystic ovary syndrome (Joffe, Cohen, et al. 2006; O'Donovan, Kusumakar, et al. 2002).

Lithium can also cause fetal harm. Ebstein's anomaly, a rare defect in the tricuspid valve, can occur at up to 6-20 times the baseline risk, rising to 1:1000 with lithium exposure. Previously, this risk was thought to be much higher. For a more complete discussion of pregnancy risks of psychiatric medications, students and clinicians should refer to the 2008 Practice Bulletin of the American College of Obstetrics and Gynecology (ACOG 2008).

Carbamazepine is an anticonvulsant that can enhance Na+ channel inactivation, thereby blocking action potentials and repetitive neuronal firing (Nestler, Hyman, et al. 2009). It is also thought to inhibit a process known as 'kindling'—a process whereby repeated subthreshold electrical stimuli can lead to the development of spontaneous seizures. Hypothetically, subthreshold environmental stimuli or prior manias can similarly kindle the development and frequency of further manias (Post, Uhde et al. 1982; Post 1990).

Carbamazepine has efficacy in the treatment of manic (Weisler, Kalali, et al. 2004; Weisler, Keck, et al. 2005), but probably not depressive episodes (Ansari and Osser 2010) associated with bipolar disorder. Serum levels of 4-12 mcg/mL may be therapeutic. Side effects such as dizziness, ataxia and gastrointestinal symptoms prohibit the use of loading strategies. Thrombocytopenia, leukopenia, aplastic anemia, hyponatremia, and dangerous rash may also develop with carbamazepine therapy. Another factor that significantly limits treatment with carbamazepine, especially in severe mania when concurrent antipsychotics may be necessary, is its propensity to induce the potency of multiple hepatic enzymes (e.g., CYP1A2, CYP2C9, CYP2C19, CYP3A4) that metabolize these drugs. It can therefore decrease the serum levels of other concurrently administered drugs and render them less effective. Notably, the antiepileptic drugs **phenobarbital**, **phenytoin**, and **primidone** also have similarly broad hepatic enzyme induction capacities (Perucca 2006). Teratogenic effects of carbamazepine are almost comparable in severity to those of valproate (Cohen 2007; Viguera, Koukopoulos, et al. 2007) so it should also be avoided in women of child-bearing potential.

Oxcarbazepine, a derivative of carbamazepine, may also have efficacy in the treatment of acute mania (Ghaemi, Berv, et al. 2003; Pratoomsri, Yatham, et al. 2006; Kakkar, Rehan et al. 2009). Serum levels are not routinely followed during administration, and there is less enzymatic induction with oxcarbazepine, thereby reducing the risk of drug-drug interactions. Hyponatremia, however, remains a concern (Ortenzi, Paggi, et al. 2008). Overall, there are insufficient efficacy data from available studies to recommend oxcarbazepine as an effective mood stabilizer (Vasudev, Macritchie et al. 2011).

Lamotrigine is an anticonvulsant that may inhibit the release of the excitatory amino acid glutamate, but its mechanism of action is not fully known. In bipolar disorder it is often used (but not FDA approved) for the treatment of acute bipolar depression; the effect however seems to be modest. Four out of five studies failed to show separation from placebo (Calabrese, Bowden, et al. 1999; Calabrese, Huffman, et al. 2008), although a meta-analysis of these studies showed an overall effect size of 0.3 (considered a weak effect size) but greater separation from placebo in more severely depressed patients (Geddes, Calabrese et al. 2009). Lamotrigine is effective and FDA approved as maintenance therapy for depressive episodes in bipolar disorder (Bowden, Calabrese, et al. 2003; Calabrese, Bowden, et al. 2003; Licht, Nielsen et al. 2010). Although lamotrigine is generally well-tolerated, there is a 0.1% risk of dangerous rash (i.e., toxic epidermal necrolysis—Stevens-Johnson syndrome) (Calabrese, Sullivan et al. 2002). Gradual titration is required to decrease the risk of rash. If rash develops, lamotrigine should be discontinued. Lamotrigine so far seems relatively safer in pregnancy than valproate and carbamazepine (ACOG 2008; Vajda, Graham et al. 2012).

Second Generation Antipsychotics (SGAs) Used as Mood Stabilizers

All SGAs and some FGAs (first generation antipsychotics) have been found to have efficacy in the treatment of mania (Janicak 2006). Risperidone, olanzapine and haloperidol may be somewhat more effective than lithium or anticonvulsants for the treatment of acute mania (Cipriani, Barbui et al. 2011; Tarr, Glue et al. 2011). Haloperidol may be the most effective (Cipriani, Barbui et al. 2011) and may have a faster onset of action than other agents (Tohen and Vieta 2009). However, it is no longer recommended for most patients with acute mania because of having the highest risk of inducing a switch to depression (Goikolea, Colom et al. 2013) and causing neuroleptic-induced dysphoria (Tohen and Zarate 1998). Improvement with antipsychotics (e.g., olanzapine and risperidone) may begin within the first week and early responders are likely to continue to improve for the duration of the period of treatment of acute symptoms (Kemp, Johnson et al. 2011). Olanzapine, however, is not an appropriate first-line treatment for mania due to its metabolic side effects (Grunze, Vieta et al. 2009; Mohammad and Osser 2014). Some SGAs, e.g., quetiapine and risperidone, work better than lithium in mixed mania (Fountoulakis, Kontis et al. 2012; Swann, Lafer et al. 2013).

For acute bipolar depression, among the SGAs, only quetiapine and lurasidone have been shown to have clear efficacy (Calabrese, Keck, et al. 2005; Thase, Macfadden, et al. 2006; De Fruyt, Deschepper et al. 2012; Loebel, Cucchiaro et al. 2014). Both have FDA approval, as does olanzapine combined with fluoxetine. Although olanzapine and olanzapine-fluoxetine combination may have some efficacy (Tohen, Vieta et al. 2003), the effect may be less than quetiapine (De Fruyt, Deschepper et al. 2012) and concerns about adverse metabolic effects would again argue against use as a first-line treatment. Aripiprazole, which has an FDA indication as adjunctive treatment for unipolar depression, does not appear to be efficacious for the treatment of acute bipolar depression nor for preventing depressive episodes (Keck, Calabrese et al. 2006; Thase, Jonas et al. 2008; Cruz, Sanchez-Moreno et al. 2010; De Fruyt, Deschepper et al. 2012).

For maintenance therapy, olanzapine, aripiprazole, paliperidone, and long-acting injectable risperidone and paliperidone, have been found effective as monotherapy treatments for the prevention of manic episodes (Tohen, Calabrese et al. 2006; Keck, Calabrese et al. 2007; Quiroz, Yatham et al. 2010; Yildiz, Vieta et al. 2011). Quetiapine has one study suggesting it may prevent both manic and depressive episodes (Weisler, Nolen et al. 2011). Quetiapine may present a challenge to lithium as the most broadly effective mood stabilizer with the best evidence base. In general, however, due to problematic study designs having to do with whether or not these are 'relapse prevention' or 'recurrence prevention' studies, and the predominance of prevention of manic rather than depressive episodes in most studies when antipsychotics are used as monotherapy, it may be too early to consider any SGA to be a mood stabilizer by the "two by two" definition (Goodwin, Whitham et al. 2011).

There is evidence that the SGAs olanzapine, quetiapine, ziprasidone, aripiprazole, and long-acting injectable risperidone, when added to lithium or valproate, can increase maintenance efficacy for the manic phase (Tohen, Chengappa et al. 2004; Macfadden, Alphs et al. 2009; Bowden, Vieta et al. 2010; Marcus, Khan et al. 2011). In the case of quetiapine, the depressive phase was also helped (Vieta, Suppes et al. 2008; Suppes, Vieta et al. 2009). In any event, whether used as monotherapy or as adjunctive therapy added to a mood stabilizer, the use of antipsychotics for maintenance carries significant long-term risks and is best reserved for when lithium has proven unsatisfactory.

Newer Anticonvulsants

Relatively newer anticonvulsants such as **topiramate, gabapentin, pregabalin, tiagabine, zonisamide** and **levetiracetam**, which are generally thought to exert their therapeutic effects by enhancing GABA transmission, may also be effective for the treatment of bipolar disorder (Johannessen and Landmark 2008). However, when used, they should be considered to be adjunctive treatments only (for example to decrease concurrent anxiety); the evidence base is insufficient to recommend their use as primary agents for the treatment of mood disorder symptoms (Anand, Bukhari, et al. 2005; Grunze, Langosch, et al. 2003; Grunze, Normann, et al. 2001; Keck, Strawn, et al. 2006; Macdonald and Young 2002; Pande, Crockatt, et al. 2000; Vieta, Goikolea, et al. 2003; Vieta, Manuel Goikolea, et al. 2006; Vieta, Sanchez-Moreno, et al. 2003; Yatham, Kusumakar, et al. 2002; Young, Geddes, et al. 2006; Young, Geddes, et al. 2006). Older publications suggest that **clonazepam** (a benzodiazepine which has also been used as an anticonvulsant) may have mood stabilizing effects in the treatment of bipolar patients, but newer studies are lacking (Sachs 1990; Sachs, Rosenbaum et al. 1990).

Further Notes on the Clinical Approach to Bipolar Patients

Mood stabilization is frequently difficult to achieve in bipolar disorder. Although the goal is to use as few medications as possible and rely on mood stabilizers whenever possible, it is common that more complex psychopharmacology regimens are required.

Outcome studies: The Systematic Treatment Enhancement Program – Bipolar Disorder (STEP-BD) is a publically funded, multi-site outcomes study designed to add to our understanding of how to best treat this disorder. The program enrolled 4,360 bipolar patients who are being followed longitudinally at 15 sites. Some of these patients agree to enter controlled studies of a variety of psychosocial and psychopharmacological interventions. Among the significant findings to date are the following:

- Psychotherapy is effective for bipolar depression but it is a slow process. Improvement occurs in a mean of 169 days vs. 279 days in the control group (Miklowitz, Otto, et al. 2007).

- Antidepressants (bupropion, paroxetine) are not more effective than placebo for bipolar depression (24% for the antidepressants vs. 27% for the placebo in a 6-month trial). The antidepressants, when added to a mood stabilizer, did not induce more switches to mania (10% vs. 11%), but the patients who participated in this study were probably at very low risk for switching (Sachs, Nierenberg, et al. 2007).

- Other STEP-BD data did show that the use of antidepressants was associated with more manic symptoms. More specifically, bipolar depressed patients who had 2 or more associated manic symptoms, showed greater manic severity at 3 month follow-up. In these cases, antidepressant use did not hasten recovery time (Goldberg, Perlis, et al. 2007).

- 262 suicide attempts and 8 completed suicides have occurred in this patient sample over a 6-year period. Lithium seemed to offer no protective effect, contrary to data from other studies strongly suggesting that lithium helps lower suicide risk in bipolar patients. However, the patient sample clearly had a very low risk of suicidal behaviors so it was not the best population to demonstrate lithium's apparent benefit on this symptom (Marangell, Dennehy, et al. 2008).

- Antidepressant continuation, in those who had responded to an antidepressant, did not confer any statistically significant longer-term benefit. Those with rapid-cycling bipolar disorder had more recurrent mood episodes with antidepressant continuation (Ghaemi, Ostacher et al. 2010).

Further notes on the use of antidepressants: The use of antidepressants in patients with bipolar disorder remains controversial. Historically, antidepressants have been used to treat bipolar depression (bipolar II more than bipolar I) and older (poorly controlled) studies and algorithms did support their use. However, newer data do not support their use as first-line treatments. They are generally considered to have limited effectiveness and the risk of mood destabilization (particularly the risk of manic induction) continues to be a concern (Pacchiarotti, Bond et al. 2013). If a bipolar depressed patient is refractory to first-line treatments (i.e., lithium, lamotrigine, quetiapine, and lurasidone) as monotherapy and in combination, and antidepressants are then considered, the following should be taken into account (Ansari and Osser 2010):

- ECT is an effective treatment that should be considered early in the treatment algorithm for patients with urgent indications such as severe suicidality, catatonia, poor oral intake, or medical conditions (or pregnancy) that may limit the use of psychotropics.
- Patients at high risk for manic induction are not good candidates for antidepressant therapy. These include patients with (1) a past history of antidepressant induced mania, hypomania, or mixed states, (2) a history of severe or dangerous hypomanic or manic episodes, (3) concurrent manic symptoms (i.e., depressive mixed states), (4) a

history of substance abuse, and/or (5) rapid-cycling bipolar disorder.

- Bupropion and SSRIs may be less likely to cause manic switch than SNRIs and TCAs.
- If used, an antidepressant should be used in combination with a mood stabilizer.
- If used, an antidepressant should be started at a low dose and increased gradually, and the patient should be monitored closely for signs of emerging mania.
- Consideration should be given to discontinuing antidepressant treatment after recovery from the initial depressive illness unless there is a history of sustained response with continued antidepressant use (Ghaemi, Hsu et al. 2003).

Summary of medication used for each phase of bipolar disorder: Based on the material presented in this chapter, the following general recommendations are noted:

- **Mania** (Mohammad and Osser 2014): Lithium is the first-line mood stabilizer for the treatment of acute non-mixed mania. It may be supplemented by an atypical antipsychotic (quetiapine is preferred). Carbamazepine's utility is limited given potential for medication interactions and slow titration. Brief adjunctive treatment with a benzodiazepine should also be considered to help treat agitation, anxiety and insomnia while more time is given for lithium to become effective. Adjunctive medications can then be tapered off and lithium can be continued once the patient is no longer manic.
- **Mixed mania** (Mohammad and Osser 2014): SGAs are first-line (quetiapine is preferred). Valproate may be more

effective than lithium for mixed episodes. Lithium may be added as a third-line agent especially if the patient has been suicidal.

- **Depression** (Ansari and Osser 2010): Lithium, lamotrigine, quetiapine and lurasidone may be considered first-line treatments for acute bipolar depression. Combinations of these medications can be used if monotherapy is ineffective. Carbamazepine and valproate are not likely to be effective. Olanzapine and the olanzapine-fluoxetine combination may be efficacious but poor tolerability makes them undesirable for first-line use. Antidepressants should not be considered first-line treatments. These can be considered only in patients for whom the above treatments (and ECT) are ineffective or otherwise deemed unacceptable; even then certain caveats apply as noted above.

- **Maintenance:** Lithium, some SGAs, and lamotrigine (primarily for prophylaxis against depressive but not manic episodes) have efficacy as maintenance therapies. If monotherapy is ineffective, then combinations can be considered (if careful consideration is given to specific interactions and side effects). Some SGAs (see above) may have efficacy as maintenance therapies, however they are primarily helpful in reducing manic rather than depressive recurrences (with the exception of quetiapine which may protect against both). The larger concern with SGAs, however, is the poor long-term side effect profiles of some of them. Given that patients with bipolar disorder are likely to require lifelong maintenance treatment, long-term tolerability is a major factor in the choice of treatments.

Future Trends

As discussed in the chapter on antidepressants, the phencyclidine derivative, **ketamine**, an N-methyl-D-aspartate (a glutamate receptor) antagonist appears to show efficacy in the treatment of unipolar depression. This effect appears to extend to bipolar depression as well. Patients with depressive symptoms, who were maintained on either lithium or valproate, showed improvement in symptoms and in suicidality within 40 minutes after a single infusion of intravenous ketamine (Diazgranados, Ibrahim et al. 2010; Zarate, Brutsche et al. 2012). Manic induction was rare and the treatment was well tolerated, the most common adverse effect being the development of transient dissociative symptoms. It is not yet known if the positive response can be sustained. Also, chronic ketamine administration, if needed, may be problematic as it may be associated with increasing dissociative and perceptual disturbances. Of note, many commonly used mood stabilizing agents, such as lithium, valproate and lamotrigine also appear to have some effect on the glutamatergic system and this may point to a common therapeutic pathway (Machado-Vieira, Ibrahim et al. 2012).

Tamoxifen, an estrogen receptor antagonist and a protein kinase C (PKC) inhibitor has been studied in the treatment of bipolar disorders. PKC is involved in intracellular signaling and is also inhibited by both lithium and valproate (Zarate and Manji 2009). Adding tamoxifen to lithium appeared to be more efficacious than lithium alone in the treatment of acute mania in two small controlled studies (Amrollahi, Rezaei et al. 2011).

Triiodothyronine and **levothyroxine** have been studied and may be beneficial in the treatment of refractory bipolar depression (Stamm, Lewitzka et al. 2014). Supraphysiological doses of T4 may be helpful in augmenting antidepressant therapy in treatment-resistant patients. The antidepressant

effect of thyroid hormone in a euthyroid patient has been proposed to be due to modulation of the catecholaminergic system
(Chakrabarti, Giri et al. 2011).

Omega-3 fatty acids, although not novel, continue to be
considered for the treatment of bipolar depression and mania.
A recent meta-analysis suggests that adjunctive use of omega-3
fatty acids may be efficacious for bipolar depression but not for
bipolar mania (Sarris, Mischoulon et al. 2012). On the positive
side they are likely to be the most tolerable of all treatments
studied for bipolar disorder.

Table of Mood Stabilizers

Table 4 summarizes the characteristics of commonly used mood stabilizing medications (Ansari and Osser 2009; WHO 2011; PDR 2014).

TABLE 4. COMMONLY USED MOOD STABILIZING MEDICATIONS

MEDICATION*	DOSING**	COMMENTS/ FDA Indication
Lithium Carbonate (Lithobid®, Eskalith®)	Start: 300 mg po bid-tid and check serum trough level (8-12 hours after last dose) after 4-5 days (after steady state) then adjust as needed. See text for serum levels.	Check baseline chemistries, kidney function, thyroid function (TSH), ECG (r/o sinus node dysfunction); once target dose is reached, check level, chemistries, kidney function, TSH, every 3-6 months initially, then every 6-12 months; NSAIDs, thiazide diuretics, ACE inhibitors, metronidazole, and tetracyclines can increase lithium level. On WHO Essential Medicines List for bipolar disorders. *Mania/Maintenance in bipolar disorder*
Divalproex Sodium, Valproic Acid, Valproate (Depakote®, Depakote ER®, Depakene®)	Start: 250 mg po tid and check serum trough level after 4-5 days, then adjust as needed, can use loading dose of 20-30 mg/kg to hasten response. See text for serum levels.	Check baseline LFTs and CBC; once target dose is reached check serum level, LFTs and CBC every 3-6 months initially then yearly; can inhibit the glucuronidation of lamotrigine; can inhibit CYP2C9, CYP2C19; aspirin can increase levels; valproate is highly protein-bound so will increase free warfarin levels. On WHO Essential Medicines List for bipolar disorders and as an anticonvulsant. *Mania/Mixed episodes associated with bipolar disorder/Migraine prophylaxis/Specific seizure disorders (see package insert)*
Carbamazepine (Tegretol®, Carbatrol®,	Start: 200 mg po bid then check serum trough level	Check baseline CBC, sodium, LFTs; once target dose is

Equetro®)	after 4-5 days. Dose requirements gradually increase over the first month due to cytochrome enzyme induction. See text for serum levels.	reached check serum level, CBC and LFTs every 3-6 months initially, then yearly; induces CYP1A2, CYP2C9, CYP2C19, CYP3A4; itself is a CYP3A4 substrate. On WHO Essential Medicines List for bipolar disorders and as an anticonvulsant. *Acute mania and mixed episodes /Trigeminal neuralgia/Specific seizure disorders (see package insert)*
Lamotrigine (Lamictal®)	Start: 25 mg po q am for first 2 weeks, then 50 mg po q am for 3rd and 4th week, then 100 mg po q am on 5th week, 200 mg po q am on 6th and 7th week, reduce these doses by 50% with concomitant valproate, and increase by 50% with concomitant carbamazepine (see package insert for full details).	Optimal results in bipolar depression may occur if serum level around 4 ng/ml according to one observational study; valproate and sertraline can increase levels; carbamazepine can decrease levels; monitor for rash and Stevens-Johnson Syndrome. *Maintenance treatment for bipolar I disorder in adults treated for acute mood episodes with standard therapy/Specific seizure disorders (see package insert)*

*Generic and U.S. brand name(s). ** Doses are provided for educational purposes only; see package insert for dosing and other information before prescribing medications. Dosing should be adjusted downwards ('start low, go slow' strategy) for the elderly and/or the medically compromised. Abbreviations: ACE-Angiotensin Converter Enzyme; bid-(bis in die) twice a day; CBC-Complete Blood Count; CYP-Cytochrome P450 enzyme; ECG-Electrocardiogram; kg-kilogram; LFT-Liver Function Tests; mg-milligram; NSAIDS-Non-steroidal Anti-inflammatory Drugs; tid-(ter in die) three times a day; TSH-Thyroid Stimulating Hormone; po-(per os) orally; WHO-World Health Organization.

STIMULANTS AND OTHER ADHD MEDICINES

The use of psychotropics for the treatment of attention-deficit/ hyperactivity disorder (ADHD) in children and adolescents is beyond the scope of this chapter. Focusing on adults, it is notable that there has been a significant increase in stimulant prescriptions for ADHD in recent years (from 1994 to 2009). Most have been prescribed by non-psychiatric physicians (Olfson, Blanco et al. 2013).

The diagnosis of ADHD in adults is sometimes problematic but guidelines have been developed (Gibbins and Weiss 2007; Kooij, Bejerot et al. 2010; CADDRA 2011). Diagnosis is predicated on plausible historical evidence of childhood symptoms (APA 2013). This is often difficult to establish retrospectively, and when earlier ADHD symptoms are suspected, it is difficult to rule out other etiologies for these symptoms (e.g., family stressors, childhood depression, learning disorders, etc.). Nevertheless, there are adults with undiagnosed ADHD, many of whom have other comorbid psychiatric illnesses, who continue to suffer chronic symptoms through adulthood and may benefit from treatment. Others may have had a clear history and diagnosis of ADHD in childhood and as adults may need to have pharmacological treatments considered or resumed. ADHD patients can have poorer long-term social and functional outcomes than those without ADHD, and yet these can be significantly improved with treatment (Shaw, Hodgkins et al. 2012). Pharmacotherapy can help improve both the primary symptoms of attention deficit, hyperactivity and impulsivity, as well as improve social, functional and executive functioning in adults with ADHD (Bitter, Angyalosi et al. 2012). Though the pertinent evidence base is unsatisfactory, many believe that functional improvement is more strongly related to the acquisition of new skills and behaviors that have to be taught via behavioral therapies. Medications can help patients be more receptive to psychotherapeutic approaches.

Stimulants

Stimulants are the most effective and the first-line treatment for non-substance-abusing patients with ADHD. Amphetamine-like stimulants are sympathomimetic amines that likely enhance norepinephrine and dopaminergic transmission. They may disrupt the presynaptic uptake and storage of these transmitters and enhance their release—in both the ascending reticular activating system as well as in the regulation of 'top-down' cortical-thalamic-striatal circuits (Nestler, Hyman, et al. 2009). **Methylphenidate, dextroamphetamine, amphetamine salts** and **lisdexamfetamine dimesylate** are examples of psychostimulants used in the treatment of ADHD.

Assuming correct diagnosis and adequate dose, stimulants' beneficial effects on attentional symptoms, impulsivity and hyperactivity are immediate and subside with medication clearance. Emotional dysregulation and oppositional-defiant symptoms may also improve with treatment if they are associated with ADHD

(Marchant, Reimherr et al. 2011). Other improvements, such as a reduction in automobile accidents, may also be seen (Cox, Davis et al. 2012).

Short half-life formulations need to be administered multiple times during the day, but not near bedtime. In recent years multiple formulations, such as extended release, longer-acting and transdermal medications, have been developed to decrease dosing variations and pharmacokinetic fluctuations and to provide continuous drug effect throughout the day (Ermer, Adeyi et al. 2010). It is not clear, however, if differences in drug release formulations and/or dosing improve overall efficacy and outcome in adults (Castells, Ramos-Quiroga et al. 2011). In regards to adequate dosing in adults, at least in the case of the stimulant methylphenidate, daily dosing based on body weight may provide better results (Spencer, Biederman et al. 2005)—see table 5.

Stimulant side effects include decreased appetite, insomnia, and anxiety, necessitating gradual dose titration to improve tolerability. Blood pressure and heart rate can also increase with stimulant administration so patients with cardiac disease may not be good candidates for these medications. When used in healthy adults however, the short and long-term cardiac effects of stimulants appear to be mild and these medicines are generally well tolerated (Bejerot, Ryden et al. 2010; Cooper, Habel et al. 2011; Habel, Cooper et al. 2011; Hammerness, Surman et al. 2011). Possible growth retardation and the development of transient tics, although of concern in children, are not likely to be problematic in adults. Chronic stimulant use (or overuse) can lead to psychosis in susceptible individuals. Increased psychosis can be seen after just one dose (Curran, Byrappa, et al. 2004) or otherwise early in treatment. Given the difficulties in reliably identifying susceptible individuals, all treated patients should be monitored carefully for the emergence of psychosis (Kraemer, Uekermann et al. 2010). Fortunately, most cases of treatment-emergent psychosis resolve completely within days of stimulant discontinuation (Ross 2006). Lastly, medication interactions of note include that stimulants should not be combined with MAOIs.

The major concern regarding the use of stimulants, however, is the risk of misuse. This seems related to the stimulants' ability to increase dopaminergic effects in the reward and reinforcement circuitry in the nucleus accumbens. Euphoria, tolerance, and addictive behaviors may develop in susceptible individuals. In the United States, therefore, amphetamine-like stimulants are highly regulated; they are 'Schedule II drugs'-- which indicates that the Drug Enforcement Administration (DEA) designates them as being in the highest risk category for controlled substances that have an established therapeutic use. The risks of addiction and misuse have led some clinicians to be wary of using stimulants even when treatment with these medications is otherwise medically indicated. However, if the diagnosis of ADHD is accurate, these medications need not be avoided in patients who do not have a history of substance abuse. A clear risk and benefit assessment is necessary. If they do have such a history, then stimulants should be avoided in most cases. Appropriate monitoring and supervision may decrease the risk of abuse. Recent data suggest no increase in risk of subsequent abuse of stimulants when children and adolescents with ADHD are treated with stimulants (Biederman, Monuteaux, et al. 2008). Notably, there was no decrease in risk either, i.e., no protective effect from treatment. This is disappointing because ADHD is considered to be a risk factor for substance abuse; older data regarding treatment of ADHD as a way to decrease the risk of substance abuse are mixed (Wilens 2004; Wilens, Faraone, et al. 2003).

Stimulants have also been historically used in the treatment of anergic, medically ill, mildly depressed, often elderly patients. In these elderly and/or terminally ill patients, fatigue and apathy may improve with stimulant therapy (Hardy 2009). Response can often be noted in a matter of days. There is no evidence however that these medications are effective antidepressants in other patients with major depression (Satel and Nelson 1989). There is controversy regarding the efficacy and safety of stimulants to treat ADHD in patients with comorbid bipolar disorder. Only uncontrolled data are available. The largest study, a retrospective chart review of 137 adults with bipolar disorder treated with various stimulants, found that 40% developed stimulant-associated mania or hypomania, suggesting a fairly high risk to this intervention; 25% improved (Wingo and Ghaemi 2008).

Lastly, students and clinicians should be aware that **pemoline** (marketed as Cylert®)**,** a CNS 'stimulant' with an unclear mechanism of action, was used for many years and was deemed to be effective for the treatment of ADHD. Evidence about a significant increase in the risk of hepatotoxicity and hepatic failure led to an FDA warning about these risks in 1999, and the FDA subsequently concluded that these risks outweighed potential benefits (Shevell 1997; FDA 2005). Pemoline is no longer marketed or sold in the United Sates but may be available elsewhere in the world. It should no longer be prescribed given the current availability of safer medicines for the treatment of ADHD.

Non-Stimulant Medicines for ADHD

Atomoxetine is a norepinephrine and dopamine reuptake inhibitor (Bymaster, Katner, et al. 2002) which has shown efficacy in, and has been primarily marketed for, the treatment of ADHD (Michelson, Adler, et al. 2003; Young, Sarkis et al. 2011; Durell,

Adler et al. 2013). As might be expected by its mechanism of action, it may also have antidepressant effects but there are no published data to support its use as monotherapy in the treatment of major depression. Unlike stimulants, which can rapidly improve ADHD symptoms, atomoxetine requires several weeks of treatment before response occurs. Response is generally less robust than with stimulants. Atomoxetine may cause increases in blood pressure, insomnia and possible weight loss. It is not associated with abuse or dependence.

Clonidine and **guanfacine** are alpha-2 adrenergic receptor agonists which, possibly through modulating norepinephrine effect, have been shown to have efficacy in treating ADHD symptoms in children and adolescents (Connor, Fletcher, et al. 1999; Biederman, Melmed et al. 2008; Daviss, Patel et al. 2008; Palumbo, Sallee et al. 2008; Sallee and Eaton 2010; Croxtall 2011; Bukstein and Head 2012; Wilens, Bukstein et al. 2012). They may be used as monotherapy or as adjuncts to stimulants. Mild decreases in blood pressure and heart rate can be seen in both. Although the evidence is based on studies in children and these medicines have not been specifically studied in adults for ADHD symptom resolution, it is reasonable that they be considered in adults when alternatives to stimulants are needed.

In adults, other agents with noradrenergic and/or dopaminergic effects may be helpful in the treatment of ADHD symptoms, although again response is generally weaker than that expected from stimulants (Meszaros, Czobor, et al. 2007). These include **bupropion** (Wilens, Spencer, et al. 2001; Maneeton, Maneeton et al. 2011), **tricyclic antidepressants** (especially the more noradrenergic **desipramine** and **nortriptyline**) (Higgins 1999; Prince, Wilens, et al. 2000; Wilens, Biederman, et al. 1996), the SNRIs **venlafaxine** and **duloxetine** (Popper 1997; Mahmoudi-Gharaei, Dodangi et al. 2011; Amiri, Farhang et al. 2012), **modafinil**, and possibly its R-enantiomer **armodafinil** (wakefulness-promoting drugs with an unknown mechanism of action) (Biederman, Swanson, et al. 2006).

Further Notes on the Treatment of ADHD

As noted above, uncertainties regarding accurate diagnosis and treatment- emergent risks can influence the decision of whether or not to treat adult ADHD patients with stimulants. In a challenging subgroup of adults, namely college students, the processes of first identifying those with true ADHD and then performing an appropriate treatment risk/benefit analysis can be particularly difficult. Clinicians should be aware of the following caveats when considering the diagnosis and treatment of college students with ADHD:

1. The prevalence of ADHD is estimated to be 5.9-7.1% in children and adolescents, and 2-8% in college students (DuPaul, Weyandt et al. 2009; Green and Rabiner 2012; Willcutt 2012). These college student estimates however are mostly based on self-report measures and not based on comprehensive evaluations of representative samples. It is reasonable to assume that the prevalence would be lower if strict diagnostic criteria are applied (e.g., presence of sufficient symptomatology, early onset of symptoms, impairment in multiple domains) and if the assessment involves third party corroboration and the ruling out of other contributing disorders. It is important to keep in mind that diagnostic criteria for ADHD are not yet well established for adults and self-reporting of symptoms alone may not be sufficient for a diagnosis of ADHD (McGough and Barkley 2004; DuPaul, Weyandt et al. 2009; Green and Rabiner 2012).

2. The self-report of subjective improvements in cognitive functioning with past stimulant use also does not, by itself, confirm the presence of ADHD. Healthy adults given stimulants may perceive and report subjective cognitive enhancements even when these perceived improvements are not confirmed by objective measures (Ilieva, Boland et al. 2013).

3. Even though a subgroup of cocaine abusers may have ADHD, the self-reported experience of a paradoxical 'calming' effect from past cocaine use is *not* pathognomonic of ADHD. There is no published evidence suggesting a correlation between this paradoxical reaction to cocaine and the diagnosis of ADHD.

4. Malingering, in order to obtain prescriptions for stimulants (for example by feigning or exaggerating symptoms), is not uncommon among college students and may occur in up to 50% of students presenting with ADHD symptoms (Green and Rabiner 2012). Also, it is difficult to identify which of the students seeking care are malingerers.

5. There is a dearth of double blind, placebo-controlled studies investigating the efficacy of stimulants in college students with ADHD. The one available small study is of short duration and does not assess academic outcomes (which are often the ostensible reasons for students asking for stimulants in the first place) (Dupaul, Weyandt et al. 2012; Green and Rabiner 2012).

6. The percentage of ADHD students who have diverted (shared or sold) their ADHD medications at least once in their lifetime may be above 60% (Garnier, Arria et al. 2010).

In summary, caution should be used when considering stimulants for college students with ADHD. As for all patients, a comprehensive assessment should be performed before treatment is initiated. In addition to relying on direct observation, clinicians should attempt to elicit DSM supported criteria and symptomatology, clarify past history of symptoms, corroborate present and past history with parents or others close to the patient, and obtain objective functional records or other cognitive testing when available. Although corroboration of history by significant others is not always possible or practical when evaluating adults with ADHD, it may be of significant value for arriving at an appropriate diagnosis (especially if the patient's reliability as an informant is in question). During treatment, clinicians should make every effort to reduce the risk of medication misuse before prescribing stimulants. The establishment of a therapeutic alliance with the patient, and more concretely the use of treatment contracts, and close monitoring, may be helpful in this regard—here again, enlisting the alliance of a family member could be invaluable. To reduce risks, non-stimulant medicines can be considered as alternatives to stimulants when necessary (even though the non-stimulants may be admittedly less effective). Finally, non-pharmacological treatments, such as CBT, should be considered for treating adult ADHD (although CBT may be more effective in combination with medications) (Mongia and Hechtman 2012).

Table of ADHD Medications

Table 5 summarizes the characteristics of selected ADHD medications (Ansari and Osser, 2009; PDR 2014). Antidepressants used in the treatment of ADHD are listed in Table 1.

TABLE 5. SELECTED ADHD MEDICATIONS

MEDICATION*	DOSING**	COMMENTS/*FDA Indications*
Methylphenidate (Stimulant) (Ritalin®, Ritalin LA®, Ritalin SR®, Concerta®, Daytrana®, Metadate CD®, Metadate ER®, Methylin®, Quillivant XR®) And Dexmethylphenidate (Focalin®, Focalin XR®)	For Ritalin: Start: 5 mg po bid (morning and afternoon) and increase weekly by 10 mg/day, divide bid or tid with last dose not after 6 pm, maximum 60 mg/day with bid-tid dosing. (See package insert for other formulations). However, the best results in adults have been found with doses of 1.0-1.3 mg/kg/day (see text).	Carries risk of abuse; may decrease appetite and cause insomnia, may cause psychosis. Avoid if significant cardiac problems are present. Monitor blood pressure and heart rate. *Treatment of ADHD and narcolepsy*
Amphetamine salts (Stimulant) (Adderall®, Adderall XR®)	For Adderall: Start: 5 mg po q am and increase weekly by 5 mg/day, maximum 60 mg/day with bid dosing (morning and afternoon). (See package insert for XR formulation).	Carries risk of abuse; may decrease appetite and cause insomnia, may cause psychosis. Avoid if significant cardiovascular disease is present. Monitor blood pressure and heart rate. *Treatment of ADHD and narcolepsy*
Dextroamphetamine (Stimulant) (Dexedrine®, DextroStat®, Procentra®)	For Dexedrine: Start: 5 mg po q am and increase weekly by 10 mg/day, maximum 40 mg/day with bid dosing (morning and afternoon). (See package insert for other formulations).	Carries risk of abuse; may decrease appetite and cause insomnia, may cause psychosis. Avoid if significant cardiovascular disease is present. Monitor blood pressure and heart rate. *Treatment of ADHD and narcolepsy*

Lisdexamfetamine dimesylate (Stimulant) (Vyvanse®)	Start : 30 mg po q am. May adjust in 10 mg/day increments at weekly intervals. Max 70 mg/day.	Pro-drug of dextroamphetamine. Carries risk of abuse; may decrease appetite and cause insomnia, may cause psychosis. Avoid if significant cardiovascular disease is present. Monitor blood pressure and heart rate. *Treatment of ADHD*
Atomoxetine (Selective Norepinephrine Reuptake Inhibitor) (Strattera®)	Start: 40 mg po q am or divided bid (morning and afternoon), after 3 days increase to 80 mg/day, maximum 100 mg/day, reduced dosing with hepatic insufficiency	No risk of abuse; slower response than with stimulants; CYP2D6 substrate. Monitor for treatment-emergent suicidality. *Treatment of ADHD*
Clonidine Extended Release (Alpha 2 agonist) (Kapvay®)	Adult dosing unclear. However may start at 0.1 mg po qhs then increase to 0.1 mg po bid. Uptitrate slowly if needed. Max dose 0.4 mg/day.	Extended release formulation. Non-extended release tablets and extended release transdermal patch indicated for the treatment of hypertension. Monitor for low blood pressure and heart rate. May potentiate other sedating medications. *Treatment of ADHD as monotherapy and as an adjunct to a stimulant*
Guanfacine Extended Release (Alpha 2A agonist) (Intuniv®)	Adult dosing unclear. However may start at 1 mg po q am or qhs. Adjust by 1 mg/day in weekly intervals. Max dose is 4 mg/day. Reduce dose if with renal/hepatic insufficiency. (See package insert for weight-based dosing).	Extended release. Non-extended release given for hypertension. Monitor for low blood pressure and heart rate. May potentiate other sedating medications. CYP3A4 substrate. *Treatment of ADHD as monotherapy and as adjunct*

		to a stimulant

*Generic and U.S. brand name(s). ** Doses are provided for educational purposes only; see package insert for dosing and other information before prescribing medications. All doses listed here are for use in adults, not for children. Dosing should be adjusted downwards ('start low, go slow' strategy) for the elderly and/or the medically compromised. Abbreviations: ADHD-Attention Deficit/Hyperactivity Disorder; bid-(bis in die) twice a day; CYP-Cytochrome P450 enzyme; mg-milligram; po-(per os) orally; tid-(ter in die) three times a day; q-(quaque) every.

TREATMENTS FOR SUBSTANCE USE DISORDERS

The past few decades have seen a dramatic increase in the number of pharmacological options available for the treatment of substance use disorders. Pharmacotherapeutic treatments are now available for the treatment of opioid, alcohol, and nicotine use disorders, and medications have been investigated for treating individuals using cocaine and other stimulants (Kranzler 2014). Detailed algorithms for the use of pharmacotherapy in these disorders are available—e.g., through the International Psychopharmacology Algorithm Project (www.ipap.org); their opiate and alcohol use disorders algorithms were updated in September 2013.

Clinicians should consider the use of available pharmacotherapies if a patient has been unable to maintain sobriety on his or her own. However, in treating patients with substance use, the beneficial effects of psychosocial interventions should not be overlooked (Dutra, Stathopoulou, et al. 2008). In fact, pharmacological interventions should be considered as only one part of a multifaceted treatment plan for the treatment of substance use disorders.

Pharmacological treatments include agonist or antagonist medications used to replace or block the effects of the specific substance used, and/or medications that may act to otherwise reduce the likelihood of use, e.g., by decreasing cravings, providing aversive reactions if the substance is used, or affecting limbic reward systems. The medical treatment of withdrawal states that emerge upon substance discontinuation are outside the scope of this chapter, but have been reviewed elsewhere (Cavacuiti 2011; Kranzler, Ciraulo, Zindel 2014).

Medications for Opioid Use Disorders

Methadone, a synthetic opioid mu-receptor agonist first introduced in 1964, is a long-acting analgesic that has shown efficacy in maintenance therapy for patients with a history of opioid dependence. When compared to non-opioid replacement therapies, methadone is significantly more effective in reducing heroin use and maintaining patients in treatment (Mattick, Breen et al. 2009).

Although methadone (at relatively low doses) can be prescribed as an analgesic by individual physicians in the United States, methadone for the treatment of heroin dependence can only be dispensed by centers registered and authorized to do so by regulatory agencies. The daily methadone dose is gradually increased over many months in patients attending these centers until a dose (of usually 90-120 mg/day or higher) is reached that stops cravings for illicit opiates and reduces incentives for drug-seeking behaviors (Faggiano, Vigna-Taglianti, et al. 2003). For each patient the dose is individualized until the desired anti-craving effect is reached; some patients may require higher doses, while others may do well with lower doses (Fareed, Casarella et al. 2010). However, doses higher than 60 mg/day are likely to retain more patients in treatment than those under 60 mg/day (Bao, Liu et al. 2009).

Methadone can cause constipation, respiratory depression (especially in patients who are not tolerant to opioids), additive central nervous system (CNS) effects with concurrent use of other sedatives, and dose-dependent QT prolongation (Ehret, Voide, et al. 2006). Methadone-treated patients who have other reasons for QT prolongation may benefit from ECG monitoring, especially when the daily methadone dose is greater than 100 mg per day (MHRA 2006). Caution should be used when combining methadone with other medications such as cytochrome P450 inhibitors (e.g., antidepressants such as fluoxetine, paroxetine and bupropion), that can increase methadone serum levels (Kapur, Hutson et al. 2011).

Clinicians should be aware that patients maintained on high dose methadone who are admitted to the medical/surgical units of hospitals for unrelated medical care are likely to need to continue their daily dose of methadone. However, high doses should never be administered without independent confirmation with the methadone center administering this drug to confirm the actual dose that the patient has been receiving prior to admission. Even 3-4 days of methadone discontinuation may significantly reduce a patient's tolerance to the respiratory depressant effects of this drug. To decrease the risk of death from respiratory depression, a single dose of methadone should never exceed 20 mg when independent confirmation of higher doses is not possible. Subsequent dose increments can then be added as necessary and as tolerated.

Buprenorphine is an opioid mu-receptor partial agonist (with very high affinity for this receptor) that is used as an alternative to methadone for maintenance therapy in opioid dependence (Fudala, Bridge, et al. 2003). Like methadone, buprenorphine is used to diminish cravings for other opiates. It is more effective than placebo in decreasing illicit opiate use, but its relative efficacy compared to methadone may depend on the doses used, with higher buprenorphine doses more likely to be similarly efficacious (Mattick, Kimber et al. 2008).

Buprenorphine treatment has the benefit of 'normalizing' patients' lives given that there is no need to visit designated methadone centers. In the United States buprenorphine can be prescribed in an office-based setting (for example with weekly counseling and weekly dispensing) (Fiellin, Pantalon, et al. 2006) without requiring daily administration in a methadone center. Buprenorphine is less dangerous than methadone in overdose with a lower risk of respiratory depression. However, concurrent use of benzodiazepines or alcohol significantly increases the risk of death from respiratory depression (Megarbane, Hreiche, et al. 2006; Kintz 2001); therefore, patients with a history of polysubstance abuse may not be good candidates for buprenorphine maintenance therapy. When used in outpatient treatment buprenorphine is combined with the opioid antagonist **naloxone** and administered sublingually. In sublingual form the buprenorphine is absorbed while the naloxone is not. When swallowed and absorbed through the GI tract, naloxone undergoes extensive first-pass liver metabolism decreasing its systemic availability. Buprenorphine is combined with naloxone to discourage *intravenous* abuse of this medication: if this combination is misused intravenously, the naloxone effect predominates and blocks any opioid effect. More recently a buprenorphine/naloxone sublingual film formulation has been developed to further decrease the risk of diversion and/or accidental overdose. However, the value of this approach has not yet been established (Soyka 2012). Sublingual buprenorphine without naloxone is available in generic form; its use however is best limited to inpatient settings where its administration can be supervised.

Buprenorphine may also be beneficial in chronic pain patients who are at risk of opioid dependence; higher doses may be needed when buprenorphine is used as an analgesic. It may be particularly helpful in patients previously taking morphine, oxycodone, or fentanyl for pain, and/or for those who have developed opioid-induced hyperalgesia (Daitch, Frey et al. 2012). It should be noted that a newly available transdermal buprenorphine formulation, marketed for the treatment of chronic pain, is not appropriate for outpatient maintenance treatment for opioid use disorders.

Naltrexone, an opioid antagonist, has recently received FDA approval in a monthly injectable formulation for relapse prevention in opioid dependence following opioid detoxification (Krupitsky, Nunes et al. 2011; PDR 2014). Prior to the availability of the injectable formulation, oral naltrexone had been available and used occasionally for opioid dependent patients if there were significant external supports and motivation to ensure adherence to this medication (Kirchmayer, Davoli, et al. 2003). Highly motivated addicted physicians and other professionals sometimes benefitted from oral naltrexone treatment for opiate dependency (Ling and Wesson 1984; Washton, Gold, et al. 1984). In others, it was not effective. The need for daily compliance with oral medication is avoided with long-acting injectable naltrexone, though monthly adherence is still required, and injection-site pain is sometimes problematic. Injectable naltrexone may be more efficacious than oral naltrexone, especially when the former is combined with psychosocial interventions (Brooks, Comer et al. 2010).

Subcutaneous slow-release naltrexone implants have recently been investigated for long-term use in opioid use disorders. Although the preliminary evidence is promising (Kunoe, Lobmaier et al. 2009; Hulse, Ngo et al. 2010; Kunoe, Lobmaier et al. 2010; Krupitsky, Zvartau et al. 2012), this formulation is not yet approved by the FDA for use in the United States.

Medications for Alcohol Use Disorders

Disulfiram, one of the earliest treatments developed for substance use disorders, acts by producing unpleasant physical effects if alcohol is concurrently consumed. It disrupts ethanol metabolism by irreversibly inhibiting aldehyde dehydrogenase, thereby leading to a significant accumulation of the ethanol metabolite acetaldehyde which is associated with severely unpleasant adverse effects (and cardiac stress). Although there is no evidence that it helps maintain abstinence over the long run, it may be useful as a disincentive to ethanol use in the short term (Suh, Pettinati, et al. 2006). It retains its effect on aldehyde dehydrogenase for up to 2 weeks, so even if the patient stops taking disulfiram and plans to drink, there may be time to reconsider and enlist other supportive mechanisms to maintain sobriety before it loses effectiveness. Supervised treatment (i.e., ensuring intake) plays a major role in disulfiram's short-term effectiveness (Jorgensen, Pedersen et al. 2011; Petrov, Krogh et al. 2011). Ultimately however, most patients who wish to drink do so by discontinuing disulfiram, and many drink while still on it, placing themselves at severe risk. Therefore, like all pharmacotherapies for ethanol dependence, external supports (such as family supervision of medication adherence) and nonpharmacological therapies (such as ongoing counseling and behavioral therapies) are needed for continued effectiveness (Hughes and Cook 1997;

Lingford-Hughes, Welch, et al. 2004). Notably, a randomized comparison of disulfiram with the anti-craving medications naltrexone and acamprosate (discussed below) in 243 patients, all of whom received brief cognitive-behavioral psychotherapy, showed disulfiram to be more advantageous than the other agents (Laaksonen, Koski-Jannes, et al. 2008). Another retrospective comparative study of 353 patients found supervised disulfiram to be more effective than acamprosate, especially in patients with longer duration of alcohol use (Diehl, Ulmer et al. 2010).

Patients who are beginning disulfiram treatment should be informed of possible medication interactions and the need for avoidance of alcohol in foods (e.g., sauces), topical preparations (e.g., perfumes), and mouthwashes. Disulfiram is not recommended for patients with cardiac disease, significant liver disease, peripheral neuropathy or psychosis.

Acamprosate may increase the number of abstinence days and decrease overall alcohol consumption long-term in alcohol dependent patients (Sass, Soyka, et al. 1996; Whitworth, Fischer, et al. 1996; Kranzler and Van Kirk 2001; Mann, Lehert, et al. 2004; Boothby and Doering 2005). Although acamprosate may reduce drinking, its overall clinical effect is relatively modest (Rosner, Hackl-Herrwerth et al. 2010). Its mechanism of action is unclear although it is thought to involve the enhancement of GABA transmission and possibly the antagonism of the excitatory neurotransmitter glutamate (Littleton and Zieglgansberger 2003). It is generally well-tolerated, with mild GI symptoms (e.g., diarrhea) as the most commonly seen adverse effects. It is renally excreted (and therefore patients who are renally impaired will need dose adjustments) and may be administered to patients with liver disease. Evidence from a large multicenter study, however, has shed doubt on the effectiveness of acamprosate (Anton, O'Malley, et al. 2006)—see below.

Naltrexone, as noted in the discussion of opiate use disorders, is an opioid receptor antagonist. Alcohol can increase the release of endogenous opioids in the brain which may contribute to its euphoric effects. Naltrexone may reduce this opioid-mediated aspect of alcohol's reinforcing properties, and modestly reduce alcohol use in dependent patients (Srisurapanont and Jarusuraisin 2005; Anton 2008). It appears to be most beneficial in severe alcoholics (Pettinati, O'Brien, et al. 2006) and in alcoholics who smoke (Fucito, Park et al. 2012). As noted, a long-acting (i.e., every 4 weeks) injectable preparation is also available (Garbutt, Kranzler, et al. 2005; O'Malley, Garbutt, et al. 2007) and, like oral naltrexone, appears to be efficacious in severe alcoholics (Pettinati, Silverman et al. 2011). Both can be helpful in abstinent and non-abstinent patients (who do not require medical withdrawal). Naltrexone may cause mild GI symptoms and infrequent transaminitis that requires monitoring. Patients on naltrexone must not be given opiates for pain management: overdose and death can result from the high opiate doses that may be administered to attempt to override the effect of naltrexone.

Some studies have suggested superior efficacy of naltrexone as compared to acamprosate (Rubio, Jimenez-Arriero, et al. 2001; Anton, O'Malley, et al. 2006; Morley, Teesson, et al. 2006). The U.S. government-sponsored COMBINE study which compared naltrexone vs. acamprosate vs. the combination of the two, all combined with medical management (i.e., brief meetings with a healthcare provider in a primary care setting), found naltrexone to be more effective than acamprosate. It also found that the meetings with a healthcare provider increased the likelihood of abstinence (Anton, O'Malley, et al. 2006). It should be noted that the dose of naltrexone used in this study was twice the usual dose (100 mg/day vs. 50 mg/day). Individuals with a specific polymorphism of the mu-opioid receptor gene (OPRM1), i.e., individuals with an Asp40 allele—coding for a receptor with increased beta-endorphin binding and activity (Bond, LaForge, et al. 1998)—may be more likely to respond to naltrexone (Anton, Oroszi, et al. 2008).

Other Medications for Alcohol Use Disorders

Recently multiple other medications have been studied for the treatment of alcohol use disorders. Although none of these medications are FDA approved for these indications, they may be considered as adjuncts or as secondary treatments when primary treatments are either contraindicated or ineffective.

Anticonvulsants: There is evidence to support the use of the anticonvulsant **topiramate** for the treatment of alcohol dependence (Johnson, Ait-Daoud, et al. 2003; Johnson, Rosenthal, et al. 2007; De Sousa 2010). It is likely to be more efficacious than placebo in increasing the number of abstinence days and in decreasing the percentage of heavy drinking days (Arbaizar, Diersen-Sotos et al. 2010). Also, topiramate (at mean doses of 200 mg/day or higher) may be more efficacious than naltrexone (50 mg/day) (Baltieri, Daro et al. 2008; Florez, Saiz et al. 2011). It is hypothesized that it helps reduce alcohol use by facilitating GABA inhibition, antagonizing excitatory glutamate receptors, and suppressing alcohol-induced dopamine release from the nucleus accumbens, thereby diminishing the reinforcing effects of alcohol (Olmsted and Kockler 2008; De Sousa 2010). Topiramate may also regulate alcohol use by affecting behavioral impulsivity (Rubio, Martinez-Gras et al. 2009). In recent preliminary studies, **pregabalin**, an anticonvulsant with similar GABA and glutamate receptor effects, has also shown possible efficacy in the treatment of alcohol dependence (Martinotti, Di Nicola et al. 2010;

Guglielmo, Martinotti et al. 2012; Oulis and Konstantakopoulos 2012). **Gabapentin,** at doses of 900 mg twice daily, was recently found quite effective in a placebo-controlled randomized trial of 150 patients (Mason et al. 2014). Gabapentin has similar structure and pharmacodynamics to pregabalin while currently costing much less because of its generic status. A small number of studies have indicated a possible role for other anticonvulsants such as **carbamazepine**, **oxcarbazepine**, and **divalproex** in the treatment of alcohol dependence (Mueller, Stout et al. 1997; Longo, Campbell et al. 2002; Martinotti, Di Nicola et al. 2007), but there is insufficient evidence to recommend their use as primary treatments for this indication. Furthermore, it should not be assumed that all anticonvulsants will be helpful in this regard: in a recent small open-label study, **levetiracetam** treatment actually increased alcohol consumption in half of the patients studied (Mitchell, Grossman et al. 2012).

Ondansetron, an antiemetic with 5HT3 serotonin receptor antagonist activity, has also emerged as an agent with possible efficacy for this indication (Johnson, Ait-Daoud, et al. 2000; Johnson, Roache, et al. 2000; Correa Filho and Baltieri 2013). The antidepressant **mirtazapine** is also a 5HT3 antagonist but has not been studied for this indication *per se*. However, mirtazapine may reduce alcohol cravings and drinking in alcoholic patients with comorbid depression (Yoon, Pae et al. 2006; Cornelius, Douaihy et al. 2012).

Baclofen, a GABA-B receptor agonist, has been studied for both alcohol withdrawal and for ongoing treatment (Addolorato and Leggio 2010; Lyon, Khan et al. 2011). However in both contexts, despite some evidence of beneficial response, no conclusions can be reached regarding its overall efficacy given mixed results from studies with different outcomes and different sample populations (Muzyk, Rivelli et al. 2012; Liu and Wang 2013).

Prazosin, an alpha-1 adrenergic antagonist modulating noradrenergic effects, has a few very small pilot studies showing possible effects on alcohol consumption (Simpson, Saxon et al. 2009; Fox, Anderson et al. 2012). Further studies however are needed.

Aripiprazole, an antipsychotic with D2 partial agonist effect (thus putatively affecting dopamine reward systems and counteracting dopamine depletion), has been studied in patients with alcohol dependence. Small and preliminary studies have indicated some benefits in reducing relapse and cravings, and improving subjective well-being (Janiri, Martinotti et al. 2007; Martinotti, Di Nicola et al. 2007; Anton, Kranzler et al. 2008; Voronin, Randall et al. 2008; Martinotti, Di Nicola et al. 2009) but confirmatory studies are needed. More importantly, it is not clear if the benefits of ongoing use of an antipsychotic in a nonpsychotic patient outweigh the risks associated with this class of medication.

Sertraline, a selective serotonin reuptake inhibitor, has been studied for the treatment of alcoholism. Interestingly, the effect of this medication on reducing the number of drinking days appears to be dependent on the alcoholism subtype. Patients who are Type A (later onset, lower vulnerability) alcoholics may respond positively to sertraline whereas Type B (early onset/ higher severity) alcoholics may exhibit poorer outcomes than placebo (Pettinati, Volpicelli et al. 2000; Dundon, Lynch et al. 2004; Kranzler, Armeli et al. 2011; Kranzler, Armeli et al. 2012). Similar adverse outcomes had been noted earlier with **fluoxetine** (Kranzler, Burleson et al. 1996). The relationship between age of onset and response to sertraline may depend on the serotonin transporter genotype (Kranzler, Armeli et al. 2011). In one study, a combination of sertraline and naltrexone improved drinking outcomes and depression compared to either treatment alone (Pettinati, Oslin et al. 2010).

Medications for Nicotine Use Disorders

Nicotine replacement therapy (NRT) is used to decrease withdrawal symptoms during smoking tapering and cessation and can double the odds of quitting (Silagy, Lancaster, et al. 2004). NRT can be delivered transdermally via a patch, or by gum, oral inhaler, nasal spray or dissolving lozenge. All modes of delivery are likely to be effective (Silagy, Lancaster, et al. 2004) and may increase the rate of quitting by 50-70% (Stead, Perera et al. 2012). Combining two forms of nicotine delivery, such as a patch and a rapid delivery form of nicotine as needed at key times (e.g., a patch plus gum or lozenge), may increase the odds of smoking cessation (Piper, Smith et al. 2009; Heydari, Marashian et al. 2012; Stead, Perera et al. 2012). Actual dosing and duration of treatment vary slightly for each formulation, although all nicotine replacement treatments involve setting a target date for smoking cessation followed by a gradual taper of the nicotine replacement over 2-3 months. In a review of 88 trials, success rates on 6-12 month follow-up averaged 16% vs. 10% on placebo (Silagy, Mant, et al. 2000). The Number Needed to Treat (NNT) was 17, which means that 17 patients need to be treated before one will be successful who would not have quit on placebo. These are not very good odds, so patients should therefore be encouraged to make repeated efforts to quit. Caution should be used in patients with a history of cardiac disease, especially when using the nicotine patch (avoid the patch if there is a history of serious arrhythmias, angina or immediately post-MI), although an extensive review of available trials found no evidence that NRT increases the risk of heart attacks (Stead, Perera et al. 2012). Patients should not smoke at all while wearing the transdermal nicotine patch, although often this advice is not heeded. Nausea and headaches can occur frequently with NRT.

'E-cigarettes,' which provide nicotine through a smoke-less device, are now commonly being used for assistance with smoking cessation. A large number of products have rapidly become available (Breland, Spindle et al. 2014). None have been tested for efficacy or approved by the FDA for this use and evidence is accumulating that they are initiating many people into nicotine use disorders (Dutra and Glantz 2014).

Bupropion, an antidepressant with possible dopaminergic effects (see section on antidepressants), is also efficacious for smoking cessation (Jorenby, Leischow, et al. 1999; Johnson 2010). Bupropion should be started for two weeks and reach a dose of 150 mg twice daily before the target stop date, and then it is continued for at least 3 months. The addition of nicotine replacement therapy to bupropion can increase the chances of abstinence compared to the use of either drug alone (Jorenby, Leischow, et al. 1999).

Varenicline is an alpha-4 beta-2 nicotinic acetylcholine receptor partial agonist, with high affinity for this receptor. It is the latest advance in nicotine addiction treatment and the most expensive of all available treatments. It may have effectiveness that is comparable to, or greater than that of bupropion and nicotine replacement therapy for smoking cessation (Gonzales, Rennard, et al. 2006; Jorenby, Hays, et al. 2006; Tonstad, Tonnesen, et al. 2006; Bolliger, Issa et al. 2011; Mills, Wu et al. 2012). Although varenicline appears to be generally well-tolerated, treatment-emergent mood changes and psychosis have been reported in susceptible patients (Freedman 2007; Kohen and Kremen 2007; Ahmed, Ali et al. 2013). Higher rates of suicidality have been associated with varenicline treatment than with other treatments used for smoking cessation (Moore, Furberg et al. 2011). However, in a recent re-analysis of 17 placebo-controlled trials plus a new Department of Defense data set, no evidence of adverse neuropsychiatric events was found (Gibbons and Mann 2013). This was true both in patients with and without another psychiatric disorder. An editorial strongly endorsed the findings and declared it was "time to unring the alarm bell on varenicline" and time to use it on a larger scale (Evins 2013). One should not ignore that both papers were authored by persons receiving support from the manufacturer.

Additionally, there are mixed findings regarding a possible increased risk of cardiovascular events associated with varenicline treatment (Singh, Loke et al. 2011; Prochaska and Hilton 2012; Svanstrom, Pasternak et al. 2012). Because of its cost and possible associated risks, it may be best reserved for patients who have failed nicotine replacement and bupropion therapy and/or for those who are fully aware of the associated risks and who allow close follow up and monitoring.

Finally, a randomized trial in 446 smokers found that varenicline worked better when a nicotine patch was added 2 weeks prior to the quit date, compared to varenicline alone (Koegelenberg, Noor et al. 2014). 55% were able to quit for 3 months on the combination versus 41% on just varenicline (odds ratio, OR=1.85). Side effects varied in both groups.

Table for Medications for Substance Use Disorders

Table 6 summarizes the characteristics of medications used for substance use disorders (Ansari and Osser 2009; WHO 2011; PDR 2014).

TABLE 6. MEDICATIONS FOR SUBSTANCE USE DISORDERS

MEDICATION*	DOSING**	COMMENTS/*FDA Indication*
Methadone (Opioid agonist and analgesic) (Dolophine®, Methadose®)	Gradually increased over many months at specialized methadone maintenance centers only, to reach a target dose that would stop cravings for illicit opiates (e.g. 90-120 po mg daily)—see text; analgesic doses are much lower (e.g. 5 mg po tid prn pain).	The use of prescribed opiates for addicts is controversial, but effective; not curative; requires attendance at a methadone clinic for daily administration; may increase QTc; CYP3A4 substrate. On WHO Essential Medicines List for substance dependence. *Detoxification treatment of opioid addiction/ Maintenance treatment of opioid addiction in conjunction with appropriate social and medical services/ Management of moderate to severe pain (see package insert)*
Buprenorphine/Naloxone (Partial opioid agonist with opioid antagonist) (Suboxone®, Suboxone Film®, Zubsolv®); Buprenorphine (Partial opioid agonist without opioid antagonist) (Subutex®)	Do not start until patient is experiencing moderate opiate withdrawal. For Suboxone® start: 4 mg sublingually bid-tid, usual maintenance dose is 16-20 mg/day or less, in divided doses. (Zubsolv® dosing is different—see package insert).	May be given as take home prescription by trained physicians; less regulated than methadone, but considerable street usage is occurring; Suboxone® and Subutex® are now available as generics but still expensive; Suboxone Film® is now available to decrease risk of diversion and to decrease risk of accidental ingestion by children; Zubsolv® sublingual tablets claimed to have accelerated dissolving time, smaller tablet, and better taste. CYP3A4 substrate. *Treatment of opioid dependence/ Maintenance treatment of opioid dependence and should be used as part of a complete*

		treatment plan that includes counseling and psychosocial support
Acamprosate (GABA analog) (Campral®)	Start: 333 mg po tid and increase to 666 mg po tid after 2-3 days.	Renally cleared; check baseline kidney function and adjust dose with decreased function; can continue even with alcohol relapse; concurrent naltrexone may increase serum levels. *Maintenance of abstinence from alcohol in patients with alcohol dependence who are abstinent at treatment initiation*
Disulfiram (Aldehyde Dehydrogenase Inhibitor) (Antabuse®)	Start 24 hours or longer after last alcohol use. Start: 125 mg po q am and increase after 4 days to 250 mg po q am and continue, maximum 500 mg/day.	Check baseline LFTs before treatment and after 2 weeks and then every 3-6 months thereafter. *Aid in the management of selected chronic alcoholics who want to remain sober in a state of enforced sobriety so that supportive and psychotherapeutic treatment may be applied to the best advantage*
Naltrexone (Opioid antagonist) (ReVia®, Vivitrol®)	For oral naltrexone, ReVia®: Start: 25 mg po q am after meal then increase to 50 mg po q am after 3 days, do not start until free from opioids for 7-10 days. For Vivitrol®--extended release: 380 mg IM gluteal injection every 4 weeks (alternating buttocks).	Check baseline LFTs. Do not use if LFTs are greater than 4 times the upper limit of normal. Monitor LFTs in one month, then every 6 months thereafter; available in long-acting IM form for every 4 weeks administration; give patient medi-alert card or bracelet. Risk of hepatic injury. *Treatment of alcohol dependence and to block*

		effects of exogenously administered opioids For Vivitrol®: *Treatment of alcohol dependence in patients who are able to abstain from alcohol in an outpatient setting prior to initiation of therapy/ Prevention of relapse to opioid dependence following opioid detoxification*
Bupropion (Antidepressant) (Zyban®, Wellbutrin®, Aplenzin®, Buproban®, Wellbutrin SR®, Budeprion SR®, Wellbutrin XL®, Forfivo XL®)	For bupropion extended release, Zyban®, Wellbutrin SR®: Start while still smoking. Start: 150 mg sustained release po q am then 150 mg po bid (morning and afternoon) after 4-7 days, set cigarette cessation target date 2 weeks into treatment. Use 150 mg po q am in patients with schizophrenia.	May be combined with nicotine replacement therapy; risk of treatment-emergent suicidality in patients under 25 years old as with all antidepressants; CYP2D6 inhibitor. *Aid to smoking cessation treatment/MDD/Prevention of seasonal MDE in patients with seasonal affective disorder*
Varenicline (Nicotine Acetylcholine Receptor Agonist) (Chantix®)	Start: 0.5 mg po bid for 7 days, then 1 mg po bid. Set quit date one week after this dose. Continue for 12-24 weeks.	Treatment-emergent neuropsychiatric symptoms and suicidality reported initially but now in question. FDA alert regarding increased occurrence of cardiovascular events, although not clear if risk is clinically significant. *Aid to smoking cessation treatment*

Nicotine (Nicoderm Patch®, Commit Lozenges®, Nicorette Lozenges®, Nicorette Gum®, Nicotrol Inhaler®, Nicotrol Nasal Spray®)	For Nicoderm Patch®: Stop smoking, then dosing depends on cigarette use: Ex.: If greater than 10 cigarettes/day then: 21 mg patch TD each day for 6 weeks, then 14 mg TD each day for 2 weeks then 7 mg TD each day for 2 weeks then stop, other dosing depends on formulation.	Nicotine replacement therapy also serves to eliminate hydrocarbon toxicity and carbon monoxide inhalation associated with cigarette use. Combination of nicotine patch with shorter acting formulation may be most beneficial. Combination with varenicline may be especially potent.
		To reduce withdrawal symptoms, including nicotine craving, associated with smoking cessation

*Generic and U.S. brand name(s). ** Doses are provided for educational purposes only; see package insert for dosing and other information before prescribing medications. Dosing should be adjusted downwards ('start low, go slow' strategy) for the elderly and/or the medically compromised. Abbreviations: bid-(bis in die) twice a day; CYP-Cytochrome P450 enzyme; FDA-Food and Drug Administration; GABA-Gamma-Aminobutyric Acid; IM-intramuscular; LFT-Liver Function Tests; MDD-Major Depressive Disorder; MDE-Major Depressive Episode; mg-milligram; po-(per os) orally; q-(quaque) every; TD-transdermally; tid-(ter in die) three times a day; WHO-World Health Organization.

CONCLUSION

Over the last five decades, multiple medications have become available for the treatment of patients with psychiatric disorders. TCAs, MAOIs, SSRIs, SNRIs and others antidepressants have expanded current treatment options for depressive and anxiety disorders. Anxiolytics, including benzodiazepines and non-dependence-producing alternatives, are available for the treatment of severe anxiety disorders. First and second generation antipsychotics with different receptor profiles and side effect profiles have expanded the choices for patients with psychotic disorders. Lithium and medications with partial mood stabilizing properties are available for use in patients with bipolar disorder. New formulations of stimulants and non-stimulant agents can be used in adults with attention-deficit/hyperactivity disorder. Finally, pharmacological therapies for the treatment of substance abuse and dependence disorders have been greatly expanded in recent years.

Students and clinicians should become familiar with these medications and obtain facility in using them. As always, the science and art of medicine comprise the ability to appropriately and carefully apply that which is learned in textbooks to a specific patient. In the clinical setting, pharmacotherapeutic treatments should be used judiciously: the risks and benefits of treatments should be considered so that every effort is made to 'first do no harm.' Often, 'less is more': one should employ the strategy of using one medication at a time, so as to have the opportunity to know what is actually working and not working. The goal is to provide relief and lessen suffering, preferably in the most evidence-based and cost-effective manner possible. Finally, students and clinicians should keep in mind that for many pharmacotherapeutic interventions to be successful, there must also be appropriate psychosocial support and treatment. Only then can safe, effective, and comprehensive treatment be provided.

REFERENCES

ACOG (2008)-American College of Obstetricians and Gynecologists Practice Bulletin: Clinical management guidelines for obstetrician-gynecologists, Number 92, April 2008. Use of psychiatric medications during pregnancy and lactation. Obstetrics and Gynecology 111:1001-1020.

ADA (2004)-American Diabetes Association, American Psychiatric Association, American Association of Clinical Endocrinologists, North American Association for the Study of Obesity: Consensus development conference on antipsychotic drugs and obesity and diabetes. Journal of Clinical Psychiatry 65:267-272.

Addolorato G, Leggio L (2010). Safety and efficacy of baclofen in the treatment of alcohol-dependent patients. Curr Pharm Des 16(19): 2113-2117.

Ahmed AI, Ali AN, et al. (2013). Neuropsychiatric adverse events of varenicline: a systematic review of published reports. J Clin Psychopharmacol 33(1): 55-62.

Ahmed U, Jones H, et al. (2010). Chlorpromazine for psychosis induced aggression or agitation. Cochrane Database Syst Rev(4): CD007445.

Ahrens B, Muller-Oerlinghausen B (2001). Does lithium exert an independent antisuicidal effect? Pharmacopsychiatry 34(4): 132-136.

Alda M (1999). Pharmacogenetics of lithium response in bipolar disorder. Journal of Psychiatry and Neuroscience 24:154-158.

Allen MH, Hirschfeld RM, et al. (2006). Linear relationship of valproate serum concentration to response and optimal serum levels for acute mania. American Journal of Psychiatry 163:272-275.

Amiri S, Farhang S, et al. (2012). Double-blind controlled trial of venlafaxine for treatment of adults with attention deficit/hyperactivity disorder. Hum Psychopharmacol 27(1): 76-81.

Amrollahi Z, Rezaei F, et al. (2011). Double-blind, randomized, placebo-controlled 6-week study on the efficacy and safety of the tamoxifen adjunctive to lithium in acute bipolar mania. J Affect Disord 129(1-3): 327-331.

Anand A, Bukhari L, et al. (2005). A preliminary open-label study of zonisamide treatment for bipolar depression in 10 patients. Journal of Clinical Psychiatry 66:195-198.

Ansari A (2000). The efficacy of newer antidepressants in the treatment of chronic pain: a review of current literature. Harvard Review of Psychiatry 7:257-277.

Ansari A, Osser DN (2009). *Psychopharmacology for Medical Students.* Bloomington, Indiana, AuthorHouse.

Ansari A, Osser DN (2010). The Psychopharmacology Algorithm Project at the Harvard South Shore Program: an update on bipolar depression. Harv Rev Psychiatry 18(1): 36-55.

Ansari A, Osser DN, Lai LS, Schoenfeld PM, Potts KC (2009). Pharmacological approach to the psychiatric inpatient, in Ovsiew F, Munich RL (eds), Principles of Inpatient Psychiatry. Philadelphia, PA: Lippincott Williams & Wilkins.

Anton RF (2008). Naltrexone for the management of alcohol dependence. New England Journal of Medicine 359:715-721.

Anton RF, Kranzler H, et al. (2008). A randomized, multicenter, double-blind, placebo-controlled study of the efficacy and safety of aripiprazole for the treatment of alcohol dependence. J Clin Psychopharmacol 28(1): 5-12.

Anton RF, O'Malley SS, et al. (2006). Combined pharmacotherapies and behavioral interventions for alcohol dependence: the COMBINE study: a randomized controlled trial. Journal of the American Medical Association 295:2003-2017.

Anton RF, Oroszi G, et al. (2008). An evaluation of mu-opioid receptor (OPRM1) as a predictor of naltrexone response in the treatment of alcohol dependence: results from the Combined Pharmacotherapies and Behavioral Interventions for Alcohol Dependence (COMBINE) study. Archives of General Psychiatry 65:135-144.

APA (2010). "Practice Guideline for the Treatment of Patients with Major Depressive Disorder, Third Edition." American Journal of Psychiatry 167(10, Supplement): 1-118.

APA (2013). DSM 5. Diagnostic and Statistical Manual of Mental Disorders, 5th Edition. Arlington, Virgina, American Psychiatric Publishing.

Arbaizar B, Diersen-Sotos T, et al. (2010). Topiramate in the treatment of alcohol dependence: a meta-analysis. Actas Esp Psiquiatr 38(1): 8-12.

Atigari OV, Kelly AM, et al. (2013). New onset alcohol dependence linked to treatment with selective serotonin reuptake inhibitors. Int J Risk Saf Med 25(2): 105-109.

Auclair AL, Martel JC, et al. (2013). Levomilnacipran (F2695), a norepinephrine-preferring SNRI: profile in vitro and in models of depression and anxiety. Neuropharmacology 70: 338-347.

Bachmann RF, Schloesser RJ, et al. (2005). Mood stabilizers target cellular plasticity and resilience cascades: implications for the development of novel therapeutics. Molecular Neurobiology 32:173-202.

Bajor LA, Ticlea AN, et al. (2011). "The Psychopharmacology Algorithm Project at the Harvard South Shore Program: an update on posttraumatic stress disorder." Harv Rev Psychiatry 19(5): 240-258.

Baldessarini RJ, Tondo L, et al. (1999). Effects of lithium treatment and its discontinuation on suicidal behavior in bipolar manic-depressive disorders. Journal of Clinical Psychiatry 60 (Suppl 2):77-84.

Baltieri DA, Daro FR, et al. (2008). Comparing topiramate with naltrexone in the treatment of alcohol dependence. Addiction 103(12): 2035-2044.

Bandelow B, Chouinard G, et al. (2010). Extended-release quetiapine fumarate (quetiapine XR): a once-daily monotherapy effective in generalized anxiety disorder. Data from a randomized, double-blind, placebo- and active-controlled study. Int J Neuropsychopharmacol 13(3): 305-320.

Banerjee S, Shamash K, et al. (1996). Randomized controlled trial of effect of intervention by psychogeriatric team on depression in frail elderly people at home. British Medical Journal 313:1058-61.

Bao YP, Liu ZM, et al. (2009). A meta-analysis of retention in methadone maintenance by dose and dosing strategy. Am J Drug Alcohol Abuse 35(1): 28-33.

Baptista T, Rangel N, et al. (2007). Metformin as an adjunctive treatment to control body weight and metabolic dysfunction during olanzapine administration: a multicentric, double-blind, placebo-controlled trial. Schizophrenia Research 93:99-108.

Barker MJ, Greenwood KM, et al. (2004). Cognitive effects of long-term benzodiazepine use: a meta-analysis. CNS Drugs 18(1): 37-48.

Barker MJ, Greenwood KM, et al. (2004). Persistence of cognitive effects after withdrawal from long-term benzodiazepine use: a meta-analysis. Arch Clin Neuropsychol 19(3): 437-454.

Barkham M, Hardy GE (2001). Counseling and interpersonal therapies for depression: towards securing an evidence-base. British Medical Bulletin 57:115-132.

Bauer MS, Mitchner L (2004). What is a "mood stabilizer"? An evidence-based response. American Journal of Psychiatry 161:3-18.

Bearden CE, Thompson PM, et al. (2007). Greater cortical gray matter density in lithium-treated patients with bipolar disorder. Biological Psychiatry 62:7-16.

Bejerot S, Ryden EM, et al. (2010). Two-year outcome of treatment with central stimulant medication in adult attention-deficit/hyperactivity disorder: a prospective study. J Clin Psychiatry 71(12): 1590-1597.

Bendz H, Schon S, et al. (2010). Renal failure occurs in chronic lithium treatment but is uncommon. Kidney Int 77(3): 219-224.

Bennett T, Bray D, et al. (2014). Suvorexant, a dual orexin receptor antagonist for the management of insomnia. P T 39(4): 264-6.

Berman RM, Marcus RN, et al. (2007). The efficacy and safety of aripiprazole as adjunctive therapy in major depressive disorder: a multicenter, randomized, double-blind, placebo-controlled study. J Clin Psychiatry 68(6): 843-853.

Berridge MJ, Downes CP, et al. (1989). Neural and developmental actions of lithium: a unifying hypothesis. Cell 59(3): 411-419.

Bertilsson L (1995). Geographical/interracial differences in polymorphic drug oxidation. Current state of knowledge of cytochromes P450 (CYP) 2D6 and 2C19. Clinical Pharmacokinetics 29:192-209.

Biederman J, Melmed RD, et al. (2008). A randomized, double-blind, placebo-controlled study of guanfacine extended release in children and adolescents with attention-deficit/hyperactivity disorder. Pediatrics 121(1): e73-84.

Biederman J, Monuteaux MC, et al. (2008). Stimulant therapy and risk for subsequent substance use disorders in male adults with ADHD: a naturalistic controlled 10-year follow-up study. American Journal of Psychiatry 165:597-603.

Biederman J, Swanson JM, et al. (2006). A comparison of once-daily and divided doses of modafinil in children with attention-deficit/hyperactivity disorder: a randomized, double-blind, and placebo-controlled study. Journal of Clinical Psychiatry 67:727-735.

Bitter I, Angyalosi A, et al. (2012). Pharmacological treatment of adult ADHD. Curr Opin Psychiatry 25(6): 529-534.

Blier P, Ward HE, et al. (2010). Combination of antidepressant medications from treatment initiation for major depressive disorder: a double-blind randomized study. Am J Psychiatry 167(3): 281-288.

Boehnlein JK, Kinzie JD (2007). Pharmacologic reduction of CNS noradrenergic activity in PTSD: the case for clonidine and prazosin. Journal of Psychiatric Practice 13:72-78.

Boeuf-Cazou O, Bongue B, et al. (2011). Impact of long-term benzodiazepine use on cognitive functioning in young adults: the VISAT cohort. Eur J Clin Pharmacol 67(10): 1045-1052.

Bolliger CT, Issa JS, et al. (2011). Effects of varenicline in adult smokers: a multinational, 24-week, randomized, double-blind, placebo-controlled study. Clin Ther 33(4): 465-477.

Bolton JM, Metge C, et al. (2008). Fracture risk from psychotropic medications: a population-based analysis. J Clin Psychopharmacol 28(4): 384-391.

Bond C, LaForge KS, et al. (1998). Single-nucleotide polymorphism in the human mu opioid receptor gene alters beta-endorphin binding and activity: possible implications for opiate addiction. Proceedings of the National Academy of Sciences of the United States of America 95:9608-13.

Boothby LA, Doering PL (2005). Acamprosate for the treatment of alcohol dependence. Clinical Therapeutics 27:695-714.

Bowden CL, Brugger AM, et al. (1994). Efficacy of divalproex vs. lithium and placebo in the treatment of mania. The Depakote Mania Study Group. Journal of the American Medical Association 271:918-924.

Bowden CL, Calabrese JR, et al. (2003). A placebo-controlled 18-month trial of lamotrigine and lithium maintenance treatment in recently manic or hypomanic patients with bipolar I disorder. Archives of General Psychiatry 60:392-400.

Bowden CL, Vieta E, et al. (2010). Ziprasidone plus a mood stabilizer in subjects with bipolar I disorder: a 6-month, randomized, placebo-controlled, double-blind trial. J Clin Psychiatry 71(2): 130-137.

Boyer EW, Shannon M (2005). The serotonin syndrome. New England Journal of Medicine 352:1112-1120.

Bramness JG, Skurtveit S, et al. (2002). Clinical impairment of benzodiazepines--relation between benzodiazepine concentrations and impairment in apprehended drivers. Drug Alcohol Depend 68(2): 131-141.

Breland AB, Spindle T, et al. (2014). Science and electronic cigarettes: current data, future needs. J Addict Med 8(4): 223-233.

Bridge JA, Iyengar S, et al. (2007). Clinical response and risk for reported suicidal ideation and suicide attempts in pediatric antidepressant treatment: a meta-analysis of randomized controlled trials. Journal of the American Medical Association 297:1683-1696.

Brooks AC, Comer SD, et al. (2010). Long-acting injectable versus oral naltrexone maintenance therapy with psychosocial intervention for heroin dependence: a quasi-experiment. J Clin Psychiatry 71(10): 1371-1378.

Brunello N, Masotto C, et al. (1995). New insights into the biology of schizophrenia through the mechanism of action of clozapine. Neuropsychopharmacology 13(3): 177-213.

Buffett-Jerrott SE, Stewart SH (2002). Cognitive and sedative effects of benzodiazepine use. Current Pharmaceutical Design 8:45-58.

Bukstein OG, and Head J (2012). Guanfacine ER for the treatment of adolescent attention-deficit/hyperactivity disorder. Expert Opin Pharmacother 13(15): 2207-2213.

Byers MG, Allison KM, et al. (2010). Prazosin versus quetiapine for nighttime posttraumatic stress disorder symptoms in veterans: an assessment of long-term comparative effectiveness and safety. J Clin Psychopharmacol 30(3): 225-229.

Bymaster FP, Katner JS, et al. (2002). Atomoxetine increases extracellular levels of norepinephrine and dopamine in prefrontal cortex of rat: a potential mechanism for efficacy in attention deficit/hyperactivity disorder. Neuropsychopharmacology 27:699-711.

CADDRA (2011). The Canadian Attention Deficit Hyperactivity Disorder Resource Alliance, CADDRA: Canadian ADHD Practice Guidelines, Third Edition. Toronto ON.

Caemmerer J, Correll CU, et al. (2012). Acute and maintenance effects of non-pharmacologic interventions for antipsychotic associated weight gain and metabolic abnormalities: a meta-analytic comparison of randomized controlled trials. Schizophr Res 140(1-3): 159-168.

Calabrese JR, Bowden CL, et al. (1999). A double-blind placebo-controlled study of lamotrigine monotherapy in outpatients with bipolar I depression. Lamictal 602 Study Group. Journal of Clinical Psychiatry 60:79-88.

Calabrese JR, Bowden CL, et al. (2003). A placebo-controlled 18-month trial of lamotrigine and lithium maintenance treatment in recently depressed patients with bipolar I disorder. Journal of Clinical Psychiatry 64:1013-1024.

Calabrese JR, Huffman RF, et al. (2008). Lamotrigine in the acute treatment of bipolar depression: results of five double-blind, placebo-controlled clinical trials. Bipolar Disorders 10:323-333.

Calabrese JR, Keck PE, et al. (2005). A randomized, double-blind, placebo-controlled trial of quetiapine in the treatment of bipolar I or II depression. American Journal of Psychiatry 162:1351-1360.

Calabrese JR, Sullivan JR, et al. (2002). Rash in multicenter trials of lamotrigine in mood disorders: clinical relevance and management. J Clin Psychiatry 63(11): 1012-1019.

Calohan J, Peterson K, et al. (2010). Prazosin treatment of trauma nightmares and sleep disturbance in soldiers deployed in Iraq. J Trauma Stress 23(5): 645-648.

Caroff SN, Campbell EC, et al. (2001). Treatment of tardive dyskinesia with donepezil. J Clin Psychiatry 62(2): 128-9.

Castells X, Ramos-Quiroga JA, et al. (2011). Amphetamines for Attention Deficit Hyperactivity Disorder (ADHD) in adults. Cochrane Database Syst Rev(6): CD007813.

Castro VM, Clements CC, et al. (2013). QT interval and antidepressant use: a cross sectional study of electronic health records. BMJ 346: f288.

Cavacuiti CA (2011). *Principles of Addiction Medicine, The Essentials.* Philadelphia, PA, Lippincott Williams & Wilkins.

Chakrabarti I, Giri A, et al. (2011). An unusual case of thyroid papillary carcinoma with solitary cerebral metastasis presenting with neurological symptoms. Turk Patoloji Derg 27(2): 154-156.

Chaudron LH, Pies RW (2003). The relationship between postpartum psychosis and bipolar disorder: a review. Journal of Clinical Psychiatry 64:1284-1292.

Chen G, Manji HK (2006). The extracellular signal-regulated kinase pathway: an emerging promising target for mood stabilizers. Current Opinion in Psychiatry 19:313-323.

Cheung G, Stapelberg J (2011). Quetiapine for the treatment of behavioural and psychological symptoms of dementia (BPSD): a meta-analysis of randomised placebo-controlled trials. N Z Med J 124(1336): 39-50.

Chiu CC, Chen KP, et al. (2006). The early effect of olanzapine and risperidone on insulin secretion in atypical-naïve schizophrenic patients. Journal of Clinical Psychopharmacology 26:504-507.

Chuang DM (2005). The antiapoptotic actions of mood stabilizers: molecular mechanisms and therapeutic potentials. Annals of the New York Academy of Sciences 1053:195-204.

Chung AK, Chua SE (2011). Effects on prolongation of Bazett's corrected QT interval of seven second-generation antipsychotics in the treatment of schizophrenia: a meta-analysis. J Psychopharmacol 25(5): 646-666.

Cipriani A, Barbui C, et al. (2011). Comparative efficacy and acceptability of antimanic drugs in acute mania: a multiple-treatments meta-analysis. Lancet 378(9799): 1306-1315.

Cipriani A, Furukawa TA, et al. (2009). Comparative efficacy and acceptability of 12 new-generation antidepressants: a multiple-treatments meta-analysis. Lancet 373(9665): 746-758.

Cipriani A, Hawton K, et al. (2013). Lithium in the prevention of suicide in mood disorders: updated systematic review and meta-analysis. BMJ 346: f3646.

Cipriani A, Koesters M, et al. (2012). Duloxetine versus other antidepressive agents for depression. Cochrane Database Syst Rev 10: CD006533.

Cipriani A, Pretty H, et al. (2005). Lithium in the prevention of suicidal behavior and all-cause mortality in patients with mood disorders: a systematic review of randomized trials. American Journal of Psychiatry 162:1805-1819.

Citrome L (2010). Iloperidone: chemistry, pharmacodynamics, pharmacokinetics and metabolism, clinical efficacy, safety and tolerability, regulatory affairs, and an opinion. Expert Opin Drug Metab Toxicol 6(12): 1551-1564.

Citrome L (2014). Vortioxetine for major depressive disorder: a systematic review of the efficacy and safety profile for this newly approved antidepressant - what is the number needed to treat, number needed to harm and likelihood to be helped or harmed? Int J Clin Pract 68(1): 60-82.

Citrome L, Stauffer VL, et al. (2009). Olanzapine plasma concentrations after treatment with 10, 20, and 40 mg/d in patients with schizophrenia: an analysis of correlations with efficacy, weight gain, and prolactin concentration.

Citrome L, Yang R, et al. (2009). Effect of ziprasidone dose on all-cause discontinuation rates in acute schizophrenia and schizoaffective disorder: a post-hoc analysis of 4 fixed-dose randomized clinical trials. Schizophr Res 111(1-3): 39-45.

Cohen LS (2007). Treatment of bipolar disorder during pregnancy. Journal of Clinical Psychiatry 68(Suppl 9):4-9.

Connor DF, Fletcher KE, et al. (1999). A meta-analysis of clonidine for symptoms of attention-deficit hyperactivity disorder. Journal of the American Academy of Child and Adolescent Psychiatry 38:1551-1559.

Cooper WO, Habel LA, et al. (2011). ADHD drugs and serious cardio-vascular events in children and young adults. N Engl J Med 365(20): 1896-1904.

Cornelius JR, Douaihy AB, et al. (2012). Mirtazapine in Comorbid Major Depression and Alcohol Dependence: An Open-Label Trial. J Dual Diagn 8(3): 200-204.

Correa Filho JM, Baltieri DA (2013). A pilot study of full-dose ondan-setron to treat heavy-drinking men withdrawing from alcohol in Brazil. Addict Behav 38(4): 2044-2051.

Correll CU, Leucht S, et al. (2004). Lower risk of tardive dyskinesia as-sociated with second-generation antipsychotics: a systematic review of 1-year studies. American Journal of Psychiatry 161:414-425.

Correll CU, Manu P, et al. (2009). Cardiometabolic risk of second-gen-eration antipsychotic medications during first-time use in children and adolescents. JAMA 302(16): 1765-1773.

Correll CU, Sikich L, et al. (2013). Metformin for antipsychotic-related weight gain and metabolic abnormalities: when, for whom, and for how long? Am J Psychiatry 170(9): 947-952.

Covvey JR, Crawford AN, et al. (2012). Intravenous ketamine for treatment-resistant major depressive disorder. Ann Pharmacother 46(1): 117-123.

Cox DJ, Davis JM, et al. (2012). Long-acting methylphenidate reduces collision rates of young adult drivers with attention-deficit/hyperactiv-ity disorder. J Clin Psychopharmacol 32(2): 225-230.

Croxtall JD (2011). Clonidine extended-release: in attention-deficit hy-peractivity disorder. Paediatr Drugs 13(5): 329-336.

Cruz N, Sanchez-Moreno J, et al. (2010). Efficacy of modern antipsy-chotics in placebo-controlled trials in bipolar depression: a meta-analy-sis. Int J Neuropsychopharmacol 13(1): 5-14.

Cubala WJ, Landowski J (2007). Seizure following sudden zolpidem withdrawal. Progress in Neuropsychopharmacology and Biological Psychiatry 31:539-540.

Cuijpers P (2014). Combined pharmacotherapy and psychotherapy in the treatment of mild to moderate major depression? JAMA Psychiatry 71(7): 747-8.

Cuijpers P, Van Straten A, et al. (2009). Are psychological and pharmacologic interventions equally effective in the treatment of adult depressive disorders? A meta-analysis of comparative studies. Journal of Clinical Psychiatry 69:1675-1685.

Curran C, Byrappa N, et al. (2004). Stimulant psychosis: systematic review. British Journal of Psychiatry 185:196-204.

Daitch J, Frey ME, et al. (2012). Conversion of chronic pain patients from full-opioid agonists to sublingual buprenorphine. Pain Physician 15(3 Suppl): ES59-66.

Darcis T, et al. (1995). A multicentre double-blind placebo-controlled study investigating the anxiolytic efficacy of hydroxyzine in patients with generalized anxiety. Human Psychopharmacology: Clinical & Experimental, 10(3): 181-187.

Daviss WB, Patel NC, et al. (2008). Clonidine for attention-deficit/hyperactivity disorder: II. ECG changes and adverse events analysis. J Am Acad Child Adolesc Psychiatry 47(2): 189-198.

Dawson LA, Watson JM (2009). Vilazodone: a 5-HT1A receptor agonist/serotonin transporter inhibitor for the treatment of affective disorders. CNS Neurosci Ther 15(2): 107-117.

de Abajo FJ, Garcia-Rodriguez LA (2008). Risk of upper gastrointestinal tract bleeding associated with selective serotonin reuptake inhibitors and venlafaxine therapy: interaction with nonsteroidal anti-inflammatory drugs and effect of acid-suppressing agents. Arch Gen Psychiatry 65(7): 795-803.

de Bartolomeis A, Sarappa C, et al. (2012). Targeting glutamate system for novel antipsychotic approaches: relevance for residual psychotic symptoms and treatment resistant schizophrenia. Eur J Pharmacol 682(1-3): 1-11.

De Berardis D, Campanella D, et al. (2003): Thrombocytopenia during valproic acid treatment in young patients with new-onset bipolar disorder. Journal of Clinical Psychopharmacology 23:451-458.

De Fruyt J, Deschepper E, et al. (2012). Second generation antipsychotics in the treatment of bipolar depression: a systematic review and meta-analysis. J Psychopharmacol 26(5): 603-617.

de Paulis T (2007). Drug evaluation: Vilazodone--a combined SSRI and 5-HT1A partial agonist for the treatment of depression. IDrugs 10(3): 193-201.

De Sousa A (2010). The role of topiramate and other anticonvulsants in the treatment of alcohol dependence: a clinical review. CNS Neurol Disord Drug Targets 9(1): 45-49.

Depping AM, Komossa K, et al. (2010). Second-generation antipsychotics for anxiety disorders. Cochrane Database Syst Rev(12): CD008120.

DeVane CL, Grothe DR, et al. (2002). Pharmacology of antidepressants: focus on nefazodone. Journal of Clinical Psychiatry 63(Suppl 1):10-17.

Diazgranados N, Ibrahim L, et al. (2010). A randomized add-on trial of an N-methyl-D-aspartate antagonist in treatment-resistant bipolar depression. Arch Gen Psychiatry 67(8): 793-802.

Diehl A, Ulmer L, et al. (2010). Why is disulfiram superior to acamprosate in the routine clinical setting? A retrospective long-term study in 353 alcohol-dependent patients. Alcohol 45(3): 271-277.

Diem SJ, Harrison SL, et al. (2013). Depressive symptoms and rates of bone loss at the hip in older men. Osteoporosis Int 24(1): 111-119.

Diem SJ, Ruppert K, et al. (2013). Rates of bone loss among women initiating antidepressant medication use in midlife. J Clin Endocrinol Metab 98(11): 4355-63.

Doane JA, Dalpiaz AS (2008). Zolpidem-induced sleep-driving. Am J Med 121(11): e5.

Dolder CR, Nelson MH (2008). Hypnosedative-induced complex behaviours : incidence, mechanisms and management. CNS Drugs 22(12): 1021-1036.

Dowben JS, Grant JS, et al. (2013). Biological perspectives: hydroxyzine for anxiety: another look at an old drug. Perspect Psychiatr Care 49(2): 75-77.

Dundon W, Lynch KG, et al. (2004). Treatment outcomes in type A and B alcohol dependence 6 months after serotonergic pharmacotherapy. Alcohol Clin Exp Res 28(7): 1065-1073.

DuPaul GJ, Weyandt LL, et al. (2009). College students with ADHD: current status and future directions. J Atten Disord 13(3): 234-250.

Dupaul GJ, Weyandt LL, et al. (2012). Double-blind, placebo-controlled, crossover study of the efficacy and safety of lisdexamfetamine dimesylate in college students with ADHD. J Atten Disord 16(3): 202-220.

Durell TM, Adler LA, et al. (2013). Atomoxetine treatment of attention-deficit/hyperactivity disorder in young adults with assessment of functional outcomes: a randomized, double-blind, placebo-controlled clinical trial. J Clin Psychopharmacol 33(1): 45-54.

Dutra L, Stathopoulou G, et al. (2008). A meta-analytic review of psychosocial interventions for substance use disorders. American Journal of Psychiatry 165:179-187.

Dutra LM, Glantz SA (2014). Electronic cigarettes and conventional cigarette use among US adolescents: a cross-sectional study. JAMA Pediatr, epublication 2168-6211.

Ebrahim IO, Howard RS, et al. (2002). The hypocretin/orexin system. J R Soc Med 95(5): 227-30.

Ehret GB, Voide C, et al. (2006). Drug-induced long QT syndrome in injection drug users receiving methadone: high frequency in hospitalized patients and risk factors. Archives of Internal Medicine 166:1280-1287.

El-Sayeh HG, Morganti C, et al. (2006). Aripiprazole for schizophrenia. Systematic review. British Journal of Psychiatry 189:102-108.

Emsley R, Rabinowitz J, et al. (2006). Time course for antipsychotic treatment response in first-episode schizophrenia. Am J Psychiatry 163(4): 743-745.

Ereshefsky L, Jhee S, et al. (2005). Antidepressant drug-drug interaction profile update. Drugs R & D 6:323-336.

Ermer JC, Adeyi BA, et al. (2010). Pharmacokinetic variability of long-acting stimulants in the treatment of children and adults with attention-deficit hyperactivity disorder. CNS Drugs 24(12): 1009-1025.

Essock SM, Covell NH, et al. (2006) Effectiveness of switching antipsychotic medications. American Journal of Psychiatry 163:2090-2095.

Etminan M, Mikelberg FS, et al. (2010). Selective serotonin reuptake inhibitors and the risk of cataracts: a nested case-control study. Ophthalmology 117(6): 1251-1255.

Evins AE (2013). Reassessing the safety of varenicline. Am J Psychiatry 170(12): 1385-1387.

Eyding D, Lelgemann M, et al. (2010). Reboxetine for acute treatment of major depression: systematic review and meta-analysis of published and unpublished placebo and selective serotonin reuptake inhibitor controlled trials. BMJ 341: c4737.

Faggiano F, Vigna-Taglianti F, et al. (2003). Methadone maintenance at different dosages for opioid dependence. Cochrane Database of Systematic Reviews CD002208.

Farde L, Nordstrom AL, et al. (1992) Positron emission tomographic analysis of central D1 and D2 dopamine receptor occupancy in patients treated with classical neuroleptics and clozapine. Relation to extrapyramidal effects. Archives of General Psychiatry 49:538-544.

Fareed A, Casarella J, et al. (2010). Methadone maintenance dosing guideline for opioid dependence, a literature review. J Addict Dis 29(1): 1-14.

Fava M, Rush AJ, et al. (2006). A comparison of mirtazapine and nortriptyline following two consecutive failed medication treatments for depressed outpatients: a STAR*D report. American Journal of Psychiatry 163:1161-1172.

Fava M, Rush AJ, et al. (2008). Difference in treatment outcome in outpatients with anxious versus nonanxious depression: a STAR*D report. American Journal of Psychiatry 165:342-351.

Fava M, Wisniewski SR, et al. (2009). Metabolic assessment of aripiprazole as adjunctive therapy in major depressive disorder: a pooled analysis of 2 studies. J Clin Psychopharmacol 29(4): 362-367.

Fayek M, Kingsbury SJ, et al. (2001). Cardiac effects of antipsychotic medications. Psychiatric Services 52:607-609.

FDA (2005). Information for Healthcare Professionals: Pemoline Tablets and Chewable Tablets (marketed as Cylert) http://www.fda.gov/Drugs/DrugSafety/PostmarketDrugSafetyInformationforPatientsandProviders/ucm126461.htm.

FDA (2011). http://www.fda.gov/Drugs/DrugSafety/ucm270243.htm. FDA Drug Safety Communication: Serious allergic reactions reported with the use of Saphris (asenapine maleate).

FDA-Food and Drug Administration (2011). http://www.fda.gov/drugs/drugsafety/ucm297391.htm

FDA-Food and Drug Administration (2013). "FDA Drug Safety Communication: FDA approves new label changes and dosing for zolpidem products and a recommendation to avoid driving the day after using Ambien CR." from http://www.fda.gov/Drugs/DrugSafety/ucm352085.htm.

Feighner JP (1999). Mechanism of action of antidepressant medications. Journal of Clinical Psychiatry 60(Suppl 4):4-11.

Ferreri M, Hantouche EG, et al. (1994). Value of hydroxyzine in generalized anxiety disorder: controlled double-blind study versus placebo. L' Encephale 20:785-791.

Fiellin DA, Pantalon MV, et al. (2006). Counseling plus buprenorphine-naloxone maintenance therapy for opioid dependence. New England Journal of Medicine 355:365-374.

Fishbain D (2000). Evidence-based data on pain relief with antidepressants. Annals of Medicine 32:305-316.

Florez G, Saiz PA, et al. (2011). Topiramate for the treatment of alcohol dependence: comparison with naltrexone. Eur Addict Res 17(1): 29-36.

Fornai F, Longone P, et al. (2008). Lithium delays progression of amyotrophic lateral sclerosis. Proceedings of the National Academy of Sciences of the United States of America 105: 2052-2057.

Fountoulakis KN, Kontis D, et al. (2012). Treatment of mixed bipolar states. Int J Neuropsychopharmacol 15(7): 1015-1026.

Fox HC, Anderson GM, et al. (2012). Prazosin effects on stress- and cue-induced craving and stress response in alcohol-dependent individuals: preliminary findings. Alcohol Clin Exp Res 36(2): 351-360.

Freedman R (2007). Exacerbation of schizophrenia by varenicline. American Journal of Psychiatry 164:1269.

Freeman TW, Clothier JL, et al. (1992): A double-blind comparison of valproate and lithium in the treatment of acute mania. American Journal of Psychiatry 149:108-111.

French DD, Chirikos TN, et al. (2005). Effect of concomitant use of benzodiazepines and other drugs on the risk of injury in a veterans population. Drug Saf 28(12): 1141-1150.

French DD, Spehar AM, et al. (2005). Outpatient Benzodiazepine Prescribing, Adverse Events, and Costs. Advances in Patient Safety: From Research to Implementation (Volume 1: Research Findings). K. Henriksen, J. B. Battles, E. S. Marks and D. I. Lewin. Rockville, MD.

Fritze J, Schneider B, et al. (2002). Benzodiazepines and benzodiazepine-like anxiolytics and hypnotics. The implausible contraindication of closed angle glaucoma. Nervenarzt 73(1): 50-53.

Fucito LM, Park A, et al. (2012). Cigarette smoking predicts differential benefit from naltrexone for alcohol dependence. Biol Psychiatry 72(10): 832-838.

Fudala PJ, Bridge TP, et al. (2003). Office-based treatment of opiate addiction with a sublingual-tablet formulation of buprenorphine and naloxone. New England Journal of Medicine 349:949-958.

Garbutt JC, Kranzler HR, et al. (2005). Efficacy and tolerability of long-acting injectable naltrexone for alcohol dependence: a randomized controlled trial. Journal of the American Medical Association 293:1617-1625.

Garnier LM, Arria AM, et al. (2010). Sharing and selling of prescription medications in a college student sample. J Clin Psychiatry 71(3): 262-269.

Gartlehner G, Gaynes BN, et al. (2008). Comparative benefits and harms of second-generation antidepressants: background paper for the American College of Physicians. Annals of Internal Medicine 149:734-750.

Geddes JR, Calabrese JR, et al. (2009). Lamotrigine for treatment of bipolar depression: independent meta-analysis and meta-regression of individual patient data from five randomised trials. Br J Psychiatry 194(1): 4-9.

Geddes JR, Carney SM, et al. (2003). Relapse prevention with antidepressant drug treatment in depressive disorders: a systematic review. Lancet 361(9358): 653-661.

Gelenberg AJ (2002). Nefazodone hepatotoxicity: Black Box Warning. Biological Therapies in Psychiatry Newsletter 25.

Germain A, Richardson R, et al. (2012). Placebo-controlled comparison of prazosin and cognitive-behavioral treatments for sleep disturbances in US Military Veterans. J Psychosom Res 72(2): 89-96.

Gerstner T, Teich M, et al. (2006). Valproate-associated coagulopathies are frequent and variable in children. Epilepsia 47:1136-1143.

Ghaemi SN, Berv DA, et al. (2003). Oxcarbazepine treatment of bipolar disorder. Journal of Clinical Psychiatry 64:943-945.

Ghaemi SN, Hsu DJ, et al. (2003). Antidepressants in bipolar disorder: the case for caution. Bipolar Disord 5(6): 421-433.

Ghaemi SN, Ko JY, et al. (2002). "Cade's disease" and beyond: misdiagnosis, antidepressant use, and a proposed definition for bipolar spectrum disorder. Canadian Journal of Psychiatry 47:125-134.

Ghaemi SN, Ostacher M, et al. (2010). Antidepressant discontinuation in bipolar depression: a Systematic Treatment Enhancement Program for Bipolar Disorder (STEP-BD) randomized clinical trial of long-term effectiveness and safety. J Clin Psychiatry 71(4): 372-380.

Gibbins C, Weiss M (2007). Clinical recommendations in current practice guidelines for diagnosis and treatment of ADHD in adults. Current Psychiatry Reports 9:420-426.

Gibbons RD, Brown CH, et al. (2007). Early evidence on the effects of regulators' suicidality warnings on SSRI prescriptions and suicide in children and adolescents. American Journal of Psychiatry 164:1356-1363.

Gibbons RD, Hur K, et al. (2012). Benefits from antidepressants: synthesis of 6-week patient-level outcomes from double-blind placebo-controlled randomized trials of fluoxetine and venlafaxine. Arch Gen Psychiatry 69(6): 572-579.

Gibbons RD, Mann JJ (2013). Varenicline, smoking cessation, and neuropsychiatric adverse events. Am J Psychiatry 170(12): 1460-1467.

Gill SS, Rochon PA, et al. (2005). Atypical antipsychotic drugs and risk of ischemic stroke: population based retrospective cohort study. British Medical Journal 330:445.

Girardin FR, Gex-Fabry, et al. (2013). Drug-induced long QT in adult psychiatric inpatients: the 5-year cross-sectional ECG Screening Outcome in Psychiatry study. Am J Psychiatry 179(12): 1468-76.

Glass J, Lanctot KL, et al. (2005). Sedative hypnotics in older people with insomnia: meta-analysis of risks and benefits. British Medical Journal 331:1169.

Glassman AH, Bigger JT, Jr. (2001). Antipsychotic drugs: prolonged QTc interval, torsade de pointes, and sudden death. American Journal of Psychiatry 158:1774-1782.

Glue P, Donovan MR, et al. (2010). Meta-analysis of relapse prevention antidepressant trials in depressive disorders. Aust N Z J Psychiatry 44(8): 697-705.

Goff DC (2008). New insights into clinical response in schizophrenia: from dopamine D2 receptor occupancy to patients' quality of life. American Journal of Psychiatry 165:940-943.

Goikolea JM, Colom F, et al. (2013). Lower rate of depressive switch following antimanic treatment with second-generation antipsychotics versus haloperidol. J Affect Disord 144(3): 191-198.

Goldberg JF, Perlis RH, et al. (2007). Adjunctive antidepressant use and symptomatic recovery among bipolar depressed patients with concomitant manic symptoms: findings from the STEP-BD. American Journal of Psychiatry 164:1348-1355.

Goldberg JF, Thase ME (2013). Monoamine Oxidase Inhibitors Revisited: What You Should Know. J Clin Psychiatry 74(2): 189-191.

Gonzales D, Rennard SI, et al. (2006). Varenicline, an alpha4beta2 nicotinic acetylcholine receptor partial agonist, vs. sustained-release bupropion and placebo for smoking cessation: a randomized controlled trial. Journal of the American Medical Association 296:47-55.

Goodwin FK, Whitham EA, et al. (2011). Maintenance treatment study designs in bipolar disorder: do they demonstrate that atypical neuroleptics (antipsychotics) are mood stabilizers? CNS Drugs 25(10): 819-827.

Gorgels WJ, Oude Voshaar RC, et al. (2005). Discontinution of long-term benzodiazepine use by sending a letter to users in family practice: a prospective controlled intervention study. Drug Alcohol Depend 78(1): 49-56.

Green AL and Rabiner DL (2012). What do we really know about ADHD in college students? Neurotherapeutics 9(3): 559-568.

Grover S, Mattoo SK, et al. (2011). Usefulness of atypical antipsychotics and choline esterase inhibitors in delirium: a review. Pharmacopsychiatry 44(2): 43-54.

Grunder G, Fellows C, et al. (2008). Brain and plasma pharmacokinetics of aripiprazole in patients with schizophrenia: an [18F]fallypride PET study. American Journal of Psychiatry 165:988-995.

Grunebaum MF, Ellis SP, et al. (2004). Antidepressants and suicide risk in the United States, 1985-1999. Journal of Clinical Psychiatry 65:1456-1462.

Grunze H, Langosch J, et al. (2003). Levetiracetam in the treatment of acute mania: an open add-on study with an on-off-on design. Journal of Clinical Psychiatry 64:781-784.

Grunze H, Vieta E, et al. (2009). The World Federation of Societies of Biological Psychiatry (WFSBP) guidelines for the biological treatment of bipolar disorders: update 2009 on the treatment of acute mania. World J Biol Psychiatry 10(2): 85-116.

Grunze HC, Normann C, et al. (2001). Antimanic efficacy of topiramate in 11 patients in an open trial with an on-off-on design. Journal of Clinical Psychiatry 62:464-468.

Guaiana G, Barbui C, et al. (2010). Hydroxyzine for generalised anxiety disorder. Cochrane Database Syst Rev(12): CD006815.

Guglielmo R, Martinotti G, et al. (2012). Pregabalin for alcohol dependence: a critical review of the literature. Adv Ther 29(11): 947-957.

Gustavsen I, Bramness JG, et al. (2008). Road traffic accident risk related to prescriptions of the hypnotics zopiclone, zolpidem, flunitrazepam and nitrazepam. Sleep Med 9(8): 818-822.

Habel LA, Cooper WO, et al. (2011). ADHD medications and risk of serious cardiovascular events in young and middle-aged adults. JAMA 306(24): 2673-2683.

Haddad P (1998). The SSRI discontinuation syndrome. J Psychopharmacol 12(3): 305-313.

Hahn MK, Wolever TM et al. (2013). Acute effects of single-dose olanzapine on metabolic, endocrine, and inflammatory markers in healthy controls. J Clin Psychopharmacol 33(6): 740-6.

Hajek T, Bauer M, et al. (2012). Large positive effect of lithium on prefrontal cortex N-acetylaspartate in patients with bipolar disorder: 2-centre study. J Psychiatry Neurosci 37(3): 185-192.

Hajek T, Kopecek M, et al. (2012). Smaller hippocampal volumes in patients with bipolar disorder are masked by exposure to lithium: a meta-analysis. J Psychiatry Neurosci 37(5): 333-343.

Hall RC, Popkin MK, et al. (1978). Physical illness presenting as psychiatric disease. Archives of General Psychiatry 35:1315-1320.

Hallak JE, Maia-de-Oliveira JP, et al. (2013). Rapid improvement of acute schizophrenia symptoms after intravenous sodium nitroprusside: a randomized, double-blind, placebo-controlled trial. JAMA Psychiatry 70(7): 668-676.

Hamer M, David Batty G, et al. (2011). Antidepressant medication use and future risk of cardiovascular disease: the Scottish Health Survey. Eur Heart J 32(4): 437-442.

Hammerness PG, Surman CB, et al. (2011). Adult attention-deficit/hyperactivity disorder treatment and cardiovascular implications. Curr Psychiatry Rep 13(5): 357-363.

Hamoda HM, Osser DN (2008). The psychopharmacology algorithm project at the Harvard South Shore program: an update on psychotic depression. Harvard Review of Psychiatry 16:235-247.

Hanley MJ, Kenna GA (2008). Quetiapine: treatment for substance abuse and drug of abuse. American Journal of Health-System Pharmacy 65:611-618.

Harada T, Sakamoto K, et al. (2008). Incidence and predictors of activation syndrome induced by antidepressants. Depression and Anxiety 25:1014-1019.

Hardy SE (2009). Methylphenidate for the treatment of depressive symptoms, including fatigue and apathy, in medically ill older adults and terminally ill adults. Am J Geriatr Pharmacother 7(1): 34-59.

Harwood AJ (2005). Lithium and bipolar mood disorder: the inositol-depletion hypothesis revisited. Mol Psychiatry 10(1): 117-126.

Heres S, Davis J, et al. (2006). Why olanzapine beats risperidone, risperidone beats quetiapine, and quetiapine beats olanzapine: an exploratory analysis of head-to-head comparison studies of second-generation antipsychotics. American Journal of Psychiatry 163:185-194.

Herrmann N, Lanctot KL (2005). Do atypical antipsychotics cause stroke? CNS Drugs 19:91-103.

Heydari G, Marashian M, et al. (2012). Which form of nicotine replacement therapy is more effective for quitting smoking? A study in Tehran, Islamic Republic of Iran. East Mediterr Health J 18(10): 1005-1010.

Hickie IB, Rogers NL (2011). Novel melatonin-based therapies: potential advances in the treatment of major depression. Lancet 378(9791): 621-631.

Higgins ES (1999). A comparative analysis of antidepressants and stimulants for the treatment of adults with attention-deficit hyperactivity disorder. Journal of Family Practice 48:15-20.

Hirschfeld RM, Bowden CL, et al. (2010). A radomized, placebo-controlled, multicenter study of divalproex sodium extended-release in the acute treatment of mania. J Clin Psychiatry 71(4): 426-432.

Honer WG, MacEwan GW, et al. (2012). A randomized, double-blind, placebo-controlled study of the safety and tolerability of high-dose quetiapine in patients with persistent symptoms of schizophrenia or schizoaffective disorder. J Clin Psychiatry 73(1): 13-20.

Honigfeld G, Arellano F, et al. (1998). Reducing clozapine-related morbidity and mortality: 5 years of experience with the Clozaril National Registry. J Clin Psychiatry 59 Suppl 3: 3-7.

Hsu CH, Liu PY, et al. (2005). Electrocardiographic abnormalities as predictors for over-range lithium levels. Cardiology 103(2): 101-106.

Hu SC, Frucht SJ (2007). Emergency treatment of movement disorders. Current Treatment Options in Neurology 9:103-114.

Hudson SM, Whiteside TE, et al. (2012). Prazosin for the treatment of nightmares related to posttraumatic stress disorder: a review of the literature. Prim Care Companion CNS Disord 14(2).

Huedo-Medina TB, Kirsch I, et al. (2012). Effectiveness of non-benzodiazepine hypnotics in treatment of adult insomnia: meta-analysis of data submitted to the Food and Drug Administration. BMJ 345: e8343.

Hughes JC, Cook CC (1997). The efficacy of disulfiram: a review of outcome studies. Addiction 92: 381-395.

Hulse GK, Ngo HT, et al. (2010). Risk factors for craving and relapse in heroin users treated with oral or implant naltrexone. Biol Psychiatry 68(3): 296-302.

Ilieva I, Boland J, et al. (2013). Objective and subjective cognitive enhancing effects of mixed amphetamine salts in healthy people. Neuropharmacology 64: 496-505.

IMS (2014). IMS Health. Top Therapeutic Classes by Dispensed Prescriptions (U.S.); http://www.imshealth.com/deployedfiles/imshealth/

REFERENCES

Global/Content/Corporate/PressRoom/2012_U.S/Top_Therapeutic_
Classes_Dispensed_Prescriptions_2012.pdf.

Iovieno N, Tedeschini E, et al. (2011). Antidepressants for major depressive disorder and dysthymic disorder in patients with comorbid alcohol use disorders: a meta-analysis of placebo-controlled randomized trials. J Clin Psychiatry 72(8): 1144-1151.

Iqbal MM, Basil MJ, et al. (2012). Overview of Serotonin Syndrome. Ann Clin Psychiatry 24(4): 310-318.

Ishibashi T, Horisawa T, et al. (2010). Pharmacological profile of lurasidone, a novel antipsychotic agent with potent 5-hydroxytryptamine 7 (5-HT7) and 5-HT1A receptor activity. J Pharmacol Exp Ther 334(1): 171-181.

Jager M, Riedel M, et al. (2010). Time course of antipsychotic treatment response in schizophrenia: results from a naturalistic study in 280 patients. Schizophr Res 118(1-3): 183-188.

Jain R, Mahableshwarkar AR, et al. (2013). A randomized, double-blind, placebo-controlled 6-wk trial of the efficacy and tolerability of 5 mg vortioxetine in adults with major depressive disorder. Int J Neuropsychopharmacol 16(2): 313-321.

Janicak PG, Davis JM, et al. (2006). Principles and Practice of Psychopharmacotherapy. Philadelphia, PA: Lippincott Williams & Wilkins.

Janiri L, Martinotti G, et al. (2007). Aripiprazole for relapse prevention and craving in alcohol-dependent subjects: results from a pilot study. J Clin Psychopharmacol 27(5): 519-520.

Jefferson JW (2010). A clinician's guide to monitoring kidney function in lithium-treated patients. J Clin Psychiatry 71(9): 1153-57.

Joffe H, Cohen LS, et al. (2006). Valproate is associated with new-onset oligoamenorrhea with hyperandrogenism in women with bipolar disorder. Biological Psychiatry 59:1078-1086.

Johannessen CU (2000). Mechanisms of action of valproate: a commentary. Neurochemistry International 37:103-110.

Johannessen Landmark C (2008). Antiepileptic drugs in non-epilepsy disorders: relations between mechanism of action and clinical efficacy. CNS Drugs 22:27-47.

Johnson BA, Ait-Daoud N, et al. (2000). Combining ondansetron and naltrexone effectively treats biologically predisposed alcoholics: from hypothesis to preliminary clinical evidence. Alcoholism: Clinical and Experimental Research 24:737-742.

Johnson BA, Ait-Daoud N, et al. (2003). Oral topiramate for treatment of alcohol dependence: a randomized controlled trial. Lancet 361:1677-1685.

Johnson BA, Roache JD, et al. (2000). Ondansetron for reduction of drinking among biologically predisposed alcoholic patients: A randomized controlled trial. Journal of the American Medical Association 284:963-971.

Johnson BA, Rosenthal N, et al. (2007). Topiramate for treating alcohol dependence: a randomized controlled trial. Journal of the American Medical Association 298:1641-1651.

Johnson EM, Whyte E, et al. (2006). Cardiovascular changes associated with venlafaxine in the treatment of late-life depression. American Journal of Geriatric Psychiatry 14:796-802.

Johnson MW, Suess PE, et al. (2006). Ramelteon: a novel hypnotic lacking abuse liability and sedative adverse effects. Archives of General Psychiatry 63:1149-1157.

Johnson TS (2010). A brief review of pharmacotherapeutic treatment options in smoking cessation: bupropion versus varenicline. J Am Acad Nurse Pract 22(10): 557-563.

Johnston AM, Eagles JM (1999). Lithium-associated clinical hypothyroidism. Prevalence and risk factors. British Journal of Psychiatry 175:336-339.

Jones JD, Mogali S, et al. (2012). Polydrug abuse: a review of opioid and benzodiazepine combination use. Drug Alcohol Depend 125(1-2): 8-18.

Jorenby DE, Hays JT, et al. (2006). Efficacy of varenicline, an alpha-4beta2 nicotinic acetylcholine receptor partial agonist, vs. placebo or sustained-release bupropion for smoking cessation: a randomized controlled trial. Journal of the American Medical Association 296:56-63.

Jorenby DE, Leischow SJ, et al. (1999). A controlled trial of sustained-release bupropion, a nicotine patch, or both for smoking cessation. New England Journal of Medicine 340:685-691.

Jorgensen CH, Pedersen B, et al. (2011). The efficacy of disulfiram for the treatment of alcohol use disorder. Alcohol Clin Exp Res 35(10): 1749-1758.

Kakkar AK, Rehan HS, et al. (2009). Comparative efficacy and safety of oxcarbazepine versus divalproex sodium in the treatment of acute mania: a pilot study. Eur Psychiatry 24(3): 178-182.

Kane JM, Barnes TR, et al. (2010). Evaluation of akathisia in patients with schizophrenia, schizoaffective disorder, or bipolar I disorder: a post hoc analysis of pooled data from short- and long-term aripiprazole trials. J Psychopharmacol 24(7): 1019-1029.

Kane JM, Carson WH, et al. (2002). Efficacy and safety of aripiprazole and haloperidol versus placebo in patents with schizophrenia and schizoaffective disorder. Journal of Clinical Psychiatry 63:763-771.

Kane JM, Meltzer HY, et al. (2007). Aripiprazole for treatment-resistant schizophrenia: results of a multicenter, randomized, double-blind, comparison study versus perphenazine. Journal of Clinical Psychiatry 68:213-223.

Kantrowitz JT, Citrome L (2012). Lurasidone for schizophrenia: what's different? Expert Rev Neurother 12(3): 265-273.

Kapur BM, Hutson JR, et al. (2011). Methadone: a review of drug-drug and pathophysiological interactions. Crit Rev Clin Lab Sci 48(4): 171-195.

Kasper S, Hamon M (2009). Beyond the monoaminergic hypothesis: agomelatin, a new antidepressant with an innovative mechanism of action. World J Biol Psychiatry 10(2): 117-126.

Katon W, Von Korff M, et al. (1999). Stepped collaborative care for primary care patients with persistent symptoms of depression: a randomized trial. Archives of General Psychiatry 56:1109-1115.

Katzman MA, Brawman-Mintzer O, et al. (2011). Extended release quetiapine fumarate (quetiapine XR) monotherapy as maintenance treatment for generalized anxiety disorder: a long-term, randomized, placebo-controlled trial. Int Clin Psychopharmacol 26(1): 11-24.

Keck PE, Jr., Calabrese JR, et al. (2006). A randomized, double-blind, placebo-controlled 26-week trial of aripiprazole in recently manic patients with bipolar I disorder. J Clin Psychiatry 67(4): 626-37.

Keck PE, Jr., Calabrese JR, et al. (2007). Aripiprazole monotherapy for maintenance therapy in bipolar I disorder: a 100-week, double-blind study versus placebo. J Clin Psychiatry 68(10): 1480-1491.

Keck PE, Jr., Strawn JR, et al. (2006). Pharmacologic treatment considerations in co-occurring bipolar and anxiety disorders. Journal of Clinical Psychiatry 67(Suppl 1):8-15.

Keefe RS, Bilder RM, et al. (2007). Neurocognitive effects of antipsychotic medications in patients with chronic schizophrenia in the CATIE Trial. Archives of General Psychiatry 64:633-647.

Keefe RS, Bilder RM, et al. (2007). Neurocognitive effects of antipsychotic medications in patients with chronic schizophrenia in the CATIE Trial. Arch Gen Psychiatry 64(6): 633-647.

Keller MB, McCullough JP, et al. (2007): A comparison of nefazodone, the cognitive behavioral-analysis system of psychotherapy, and their combination for the treatment of chronic depression. New England Journal of Medicine 342:1462-1470.

Kemp DE, Johnson E, et al. (2011). Clinical utility of early improvement to predict response or remission in acute mania: focus on olanzapine and risperidone. J Clin Psychiatry 72(9): 1236-1241.

Khan A (2008). Current evidence for aripiprazole as augmentation therapy in major depressive disorder. Expert Rev Neurother 8(10): 1435-1447.

Khan A (2009). Vilazodone, a novel dual-acting serotonergic antidepressant for managing major depression. Expert Opin Investig Drugs 18(11): 1753-1764.

Khan A, Cutler AJ, et al. (2011). A randomized, double-blind, placebo-controlled, 8-week study of vilazodone, a serotonergic agent for the treatment of major depressive disorder. J Clin Psychiatry 72(4): 441-447.

Khan A, Joyce M, et al. (2011). A randomized, double-blind study of once-daily extended release quetiapine fumarate (quetiapine XR) monotherapy in patients with generalized anxiety disorder. J Clin Psychopharmacol 31(4): 418-428.

Khin NA, Chen YF, et al. (2011). Exploratory analyses of efficacy data from major depressive disorder trials submitted to the US Food and Drug Administration in support of new drug applications. J Clin Psychiatry 72(4): 464-472.

Khong TP, de Vries F, et al. (2012). Potential impact of benzodiazepine use on the rate of hip fractures in five large European countries and the United States. Calcif Tissue Int 91(1): 24-31.

Kim H, Lim SW, et al. (2006). Monoamine transporter gene polymorphisms and antidepressant response in Koreans with late-life depression. Journal of the American Medical Association 296:1609-1618.

King M, Sibbald B, et al. (2000). Randomized controlled trial of non-directive counseling, cognitive-behavior therapy and usual general practitioner care in the management of depression as well as mixed anxiety and depression in primary care. Health Technology Assessment 4:1-83.

Kinon BJ, Volavka J, et al. (2008). Standard and higher dose of olanzapine in patients with schizophrenia or schizoaffective disorder: a randomized, double-blind, fixed-dose study. J Clin Psychopharmacol 28(4): 392-400.

Kintz P (2001). Deaths involving buprenorphine: a compendium of French cases. Forensic Science International 121:65-69.

Kirchmayer U, Davoli M, et al. (2003). Naltrexone maintenance treatment for opioid dependence. Cochrane Database of Systematic Reviews CD001333.

Kirsch I, Deacon BJ, et al. (2008). "Initial severity and antidepressant benefits: a meta-analysis of data submitted to the Food and Drug Administration." PLoS Med 5(2): e45.

Kleindienst N, Severus WE, et al. (2005). Is polarity of recurrence related to serum lithium level in patients with bipolar disorder? European Archives of Psychiatry and Clinical Neuroscience 255:72-74.

Kleindienst N, Severus WE, et al. (2007). Are serum lithium levels related to the polarity of recurrence in bipolar disorders? Evidence from a multicenter trial. International Clinical Psychopharmacology 22:125-131.

Ko DT, Hebert PR, et al. (2002). Beta-blocker therapy and symptoms of depression, fatigue, and sexual dysfunction. Journal of the American Medical Association 288:351-357.

Koegelenberb CF, Noor F, et al. (2014). Efficacy of varenicline combined with nicotine replacement therapy vs. varenicline alone for smoking cessation: a randomized clinical trail. JAMA 312(2): 155-61.

Kohen I, Kremen N (2007). Varenicline-induced manic episode in a patient with bipolar disorder. American Journal of Psychiatry 164:1269-1270.

Kolla BP, Lovely JK, et al. (2013). Zolpidem is independently associated with increased risk of inpatient falls. J Hosp Med 8(1): 1-6.

Komossa K, Rummel-Kluge C, et al. (2010). Olanzapine versus other atypical antipsychotics for schizophrenia. Cochrane Database Syst Rev(3): CD006654.

Komossa K, Rummel-Kluge C, et al. (2011). Risperidone versus other atypical antipsychotics for schizophrenia. Cochrane Database Syst Rev(1): CD006626.

Kooij SJ, Bejerot S, et al. (2010). European consensus statement on diagnosis and treatment of adult ADHD: The European Network Adult ADHD. BMC Psychiatry 10: 67.

Kraemer M, Uekermann J, et al. (2010). Methylphenidate-induced psychosis in adult attention-deficit/hyperactivity disorder: report of 3 new cases and review of the literature. Clin Neuropharmacol 33(4): 204-206.

Kraft JB, Peters EJ, et al. (2007). Analysis of association between the serotonin transporter and antidepressant response in a large clinical sample. Biological Psychiatry 61:734-742.

Kranzler HR, Armeli S, et al. (2011). A double-blind, randomized trial of sertraline for alcohol dependence: moderation by age of onset [corrected] and 5-hydroxytryptamine transporter-linked promoter region genotype. J Clin Psychopharmacol 31(1): 22-30.

Kranzler HR, Armeli S, et al. (2012). Post-treatment outcomes in a double-blind, randomized trial of sertraline for alcohol dependence. Alcohol Clin Exp Res 36(4): 739-744.

Kranzler HR, Burleson JA, et al. (1996). Fluoxetine treatment seems to reduce the beneficial effects of cognitive-behavioral therapy in type B alcoholics. Alcohol Clin Exp Res 20(9): 1534-1541.

Kranzler HR, Ciraulo DA, Zindel LH, Eds. (2014). *Clinical Manual of Addiction Psychopharmacology, Second Edition.* Washington, DC, American Psychiatric Publishing.

Kranzler HR, Van Kirk J (2001). Efficacy of naltrexone and acamprosate for alcoholism treatment: a meta-analysis. Alcoholism: Clinical and Experimental Research 25:1335-1341.

Kreyenbuhl J, Slade EP, et al. (2011). Time to discontinuation of first- and second-generation antipsychotic medications in the treatment of schizophrenia. Schizophr Res 131(1-3): 127-132.

Krupitsky E, Nunes EV, et al. (2011). Injectable extended-release naltrexone for opioid dependence. Lancet 378(9792): 665; author reply 666.

Krupitsky E, Zvartau E, et al. (2012). Randomized trial of long-acting sustained-release naltrexone implant vs oral naltrexone or placebo for preventing relapse to opioid dependence. Arch Gen Psychiatry 69(9): 973-981.

Kuhn R (1958). The treatment of depressive states with G 22355 (imipramine hydrochloride). American Journal of Psychiatry 115:459-464.

Kung S, Espinel Z, et al. (2012). Treatment of nightmares with prazosin: a systematic review. Mayo Clin Proc 87(9): 890-900.

Kunoe N, Lobmaier P, et al. (2009). Naltrexone implants after in-patient treatment for opioid dependence: randomised controlled trial. Br J Psychiatry 194(6): 541-546.

Kunoe N, Lobmaier P, et al. (2010). Retention in naltrexone implant treatment for opioid dependence. Drug Alcohol Depend 111(1-2): 166-169.

Laaksonen E, Koski-Jannes A, et al. (2008). A randomized, multicentre, open-label, comparative trial of disulfiram, naltrexone and acamprosate in the treatment of alcohol dependence. Alcohol and Alcoholism 43:53-61.

Laan W, Grobbee DE, et al. (2010). Adjuvant aspirin therapy reduces symptoms of schizophrenia spectrum disorders: results from a randomized, double-blind, placebo-controlled trial. J Clin Psychiatry 71(5): 520-527.

Lader M, Scotto JC (1998). A multicenter double-blind comparison of hydroxyzine, buspirone and placebo in patients with generalized anxiety disorder. Psychopharmacology 139:402-406.

Lamberti JS, Olson D, et al. (2006). Prevalence of the metabolic syndrome among patients receiving clozapine. American Journal of Psychiatry 163:1273-1276.

Larkin GL, Beautrais AL (2011). A preliminary naturalistic study of low-dose ketamine for depression and suicide ideation in the emergency department. Int J Neuropsychopharmacol 14(8): 1127-1131.

Laughren TP, Gobburu J, et al. (2011). Vilazodone: clinical basis for the US Food and Drug Administration's approval of a new antidepressant. J Clin Psychiatry 72(9): 1166-1173.

Lehman H (1964). On acute schizophrenic patients. In: Lehman H, Ban T, eds. The butyrophenones in psychiatry. Montreal, Canada, Quebec Psychopharmacological Research Association.

Lekman M, Paddock S, et al. (2008). Pharmacogenetics of major depression: insights from level 1 of the Sequenced Treatment Alternatives to Relieve Depression (STAR*D) trial. Molecular Diagnosis and Therapy 12:321-330.

Lenox RH, Hahn CG (2000). Overview of the mechanism of action of lithium in the brain: fifty-year update. Journal of Clinical Psychiatry 61(Suppl 9):5-15.

Leon AC, Solomon DA, et al. (2011). Antidepressants and risks of suicide and suicide attempts: a 27-year observational study. J Clin Psychiatry 72(5): 580-586.

Lepkifker E, Sverdlik A, et al. (2004). Renal insufficiency in long-term lithium treatment. Journal of Clinical Psychiatry 65:850-856.

Lerner V, Miodownik C, et al. (2001). Vitamin B(6) in the treatment of tardive dyskinesia: a double-blind, placebo-controlled, crossover study. Am J Psychiatry 158(9):1511-4.

Leucht C, Heres S, et al. (2011). Oral versus depot antipsychotic drugs for schizophrenia--a critical systematic review and meta-analysis of randomised long-term trials. Schizophr Res 127(1-3): 83-92.

Leucht S, Busch R, et al. (2007). Early prediction of antipsychotic non-response among patients with schizophrenia. J Clin Psychiatry 68(3): 352-360.

Leucht S, Komossa K, et al. (2009). A meta-analysis of head-to-head comparisons of second-generation antipsychotics in the treatment of schizophrenia. Am J Psychiatry 166(2): 152-163.

Leverich GS, Altshuler LL, et al. (2006). Risk of switch in mood polarity to hypomania or mania in patients with bipolar depression during acute and continuation trials of venlafaxine, sertraline, and bupropion as adjuncts to mood stabilizers. American Journal of Psychiatry 163:232-239.

Lewis SW, Barnes TR, et al. (2006). Randomized controlled trial of effect of prescription of clozapine versus other second-generation antipsychotic drugs in resistant schizophrenia. Schizophrenia Bulletin 32:715-723.

Liappas IA, Malitas PN, et al. (2003). Zolpidem dependence case series: possible neurobiological mechanisms and clinical management. Journal of Psychopharmacology 17:131-135.

Licht RW, Nielsen JN, et al. (2010). Lamotrigine versus lithium as maintenance treatment in bipolar I disorder: an open, randomized effectiveness study mimicking clinical practice. The 6th trial of the Danish University Antidepressant Group (DUAG-6). Bipolar Disord 12(5): 483-493.

Lieberman JA, Stroup TS, et al. (2005). Effectiveness of antipsychotic drugs in patients with chronic schizophrenia. New England Journal of Med 353:1209-1223.

Lieberman JA, Stroup TS, et al. (2005). Effectiveness of antipsychotic drugs in patients with chronic schizophrenia. New England Journal of Med 353:1209-1223.

Lieberman JA, T. S. Stroup (2011). The NIMH-CATIE Schizophrenia Study: what did we learn? Am J Psychiatry 168(8): 770-775.

Lin FY, Chen PC, et al. (2014). Retrospective population cohort study on hip fracture risk associated with zolpidem medication. Sleep 37(4): 673-679.

Lindenmayer JP, Citrome L, et al. (2011). A randomized, double-blind, parallel-group, fixed-dose, clinical trial of quetiapine at 600 versus 1200 mg/d for patients with treatment-resistant schizophrenia or schizoaffective disorder. J Clin Psychopharmacol 31(2): 160-168.

Ling W, Wesson RD (1984). Naltrexone treatment for addicted healthcare professionals: a collaborative private practice experience. Journal of Clinical Psychiatry 45:46-48.

Lingford-Hughes AR, Welch S, et al. (2004). Evidence-based guidelines for the pharmacological management of substance misuse, addiction and comorbidity: recommendations from the British Association for Psychopharmacology. Journal of Psychopharmacology 18:293-335.

Lipkovich I, Citrome L, et al. (2006). Early predictors of substantial weight gain in bipolar patients treated with olanzapine. Journal of Clinical Psychopharmacology 26:316-320.

Lippman SB, Nash K (1990). Monoamine oxidase inhibitor update. Potential adverse food and drug interactions. Drug Safety 5:195-204.

Littleton J, Zieglgansberger W (2003). Pharmacological mechanisms of naltrexone and acamprosate in the prevention of relapse in alcohol dependence. American Journal on Addictions 12(Suppl 1):S3-S11.

Liu J, Wang LN (2013). Baclofn for alcohol withdrawal. Cochrane Database Syst Rev 2: CD008502.

Liu J, Wang LN (2012). Ramelteon in the treatment of chronic insomnia: systematic review and meta-analysis. Int J Clin Pract 66(9): 867-873.

Livingstone C, Rampes H (2006). Lithium: a review of its metabolic adverse effects. J Psychopharmacol 20(3): 347-355.

Llorca PM, Spadone C, et al. (2002). Efficacy and safety of hydroxyzine in the treatment of generalized anxiety disorder: a 3-month double blind study. Journal of Clinical Psychiatry 63:1020-1027.

Loebel A, Cucchiaro J, et al. (2014). Lurasidone monotherapy in the treatment of bipolar I depression: a randomized, double-blind, placebo-controlled study. Am J Psychiatry 171(2): 160-168.

Logan BK, Couper FJ (2001). Zolpidem and driving impairment. J Forensic Sci 46(1): 105-110.

Lonergan E, Britton AM, et al. (2007). Antipsychotics for delirium. Cochrane Database of Systematic Reviews CD005594.

Longo LP, Campbell T, et al. (2002). Divalproex sodium (Depakote) for alcohol withdrawal and relapse prevention. J Addict Dis 21(2): 55-64.

Loscher W, Rogawski MA (2012). How theories evolved concerning the mechanism of action of barbiturates. Epilepsia 53 Suppl 8: 12-25.

Lyon JE, Khan RA, et al. (2011). Treating alcohol withdrawal with oral baclofen: a randomized, double-blind, placebo-controlled trial. J Hosp Med 6(8): 469-474.

Lyoo IK, Dager SR, et al. (2010). Lithium-induced gray matter volume increase as a neural correlate of treatment response in bipolar disorder: a longitudinal brain imaging study. Neuropsychopharmacology 35(8): 1743-1750.

Maayan L, Vakhrusheva J, et al. (2010). Effectiveness of medications used to attenuate antipsychotic-related weight gain and metabolic abnormalities: a systematic review and meta-analysis. Neuropsychopharmacology 35(7): 1520-1530.

Macdonald KJ, Young LT (2002). Newer antiepileptic drugs in bipolar disorder: rationale for use and role in therapy. CNS Drugs 16:549-562.

Macfadden W, Alphs L, et al. (2009). A randomized, double-blind, placebo-controlled study of maintenance treatment with adjunctive risperidone long-acting therapy in patients with bipolar I disorder who relapse frequently. Bipolar Disord 11(8): 827-839.

Machado-Vieira R, Ibrahim L, et al. (2012). Novel glutamatergic agents for major depressive disorder and bipolar disorder. Pharmacol Biochem Behav 100(4): 678-687.

Magni G (1991). The use of antidepressants in the treatment of chronic pain. A review of the current evidence. Drugs 42:730-748.

Mahmoudi-Gharaei J, Dodangi N, et al. (2011). Duloxetine in the treatment of adolescents with attention deficit/hyperactivity disorder: an open-label study. Hum Psychopharmacol 26(2): 155-160.

Maina G, Albert U, et al. (2004). Weight gain during long-term treatment of obsessive-compulsive disorder: a prospective comparison between serotonin reputake inhibitors. J Clin Psychiatry 65(10): 1365-71.

Malhotra AK, Murphy GM Jr., et al. (2004). Pharmacogenetics of psychotropic drug response. American Journal of Psychiatry 161:780-796.

Mamo D, Graff A, et al. (2007). Differential effects of aripiprazole on D(2), 5-HT(2), and 5-HT(1A) receptor occupancy in patients with schizophrenia: a triple tracer PET study. American Journal of Psychiatry 164:1411-1417.

Maneeton N, Maneeton B, et al. (2011). Bupropion for adults with attention-deficit hyperactivity disorder: meta-analysis of randomized, placebo-controlled trials. Psychiatry Clin Neurosci 65(7): 611-617.

Mann K, Lehert P, et al. (2004). The efficacy of acamprosate in the maintenance of abstinence in alcohol-dependent individuals: results of a meta-analysis. Alcoholism: Clinical and Experimental Research 28:51-63.

Mantovani C, Labate CM, et al. (2013). Are low doses of antipsychotics effective in the management of psychomotor agitation? A randomized, rated-blind trial of 4 intramuscular interventions. J Clin Psychopharmacol 33(3): 306-312.

Marangell LB, Dennehy EB, et al. (2008): Case-control analyses of the impact of pharmacotherapy on prospectively observed suicide attempts and completed suicides in bipolar disorder: findings from STEP-BD. Journal of Clinical Psychiatry 69:916-922.

Marchant BK, Reimherr FW, et al. (2011). Methylphenidate transdermal system in adult ADHD and impact on emotional and oppositional symptoms. J Atten Disord 15(4): 295-304.

Marcus R, Khan A, et al. (2011). Efficacy of aripiprazole adjunctive to lithium or valproate in the long-term treatment of patients with bipolar I disorder with an inadequate response to lithium or valproate monotherapy: a multicenter, double-blind, randomized study. Bipolar Disord 13(2): 133-144.

Marcus RN, McQuade RD, et al. (2008). The efficacy and safety of aripiprazole as adjunctive therapy in major depressive disorder: a second multicenter, randomized, double-blind, placebo-controlled study. J Clin Psychopharmacol 28(2): 156-165.

Martinotti G, Di Nicola M, et al. (2007). Efficacy and safety of aripiprazole in alcohol dependence. Am J Drug Alcohol Abuse 33(3): 393-401.

Martinotti G, Di Nicola M, et al. (2007). High and low dosage oxcarbazepine versus naltrexone for the prevention of relapse in alcohol-dependent patients. Hum Psychopharmacol 22(3): 149-156.

Martinotti G, Di Nicola M, et al. (2009). Aripiprazole in the treatment of patients with alcohol dependence: a double-blind, comparison trial vs. naltrexone. J Psychopharmacol 23(2): 123-129.

Martinotti G, Di Nicola M, et al. (2010). Pregabalin versus naltrexone in alcohol dependence: a randomised, double-blind, comparison trial. J Psychopharmacol 24(9): 1367-1374.

Masi G, Brovedani P (2011). The hippocampus, neurotrophic factors and depression: possible implications for the pharmacotherapy of depression. CNS Drugs 25(11): 913-931.

Mason BJ, Quello S, et al. (2014). Gabapentin treatment for alcohol dependence: a randomized clinical trial. JAMA Intern Med 174(1):70-77.

Mathew SJ, Shah A, et al. (2012). Ketamine for treatment-resistant unipolar depression: current evidence. CNS Drugs 26(3): 189-204.

Mattick RP, Breen C, et al. (2009). Methadone maintenance therapy versus no opioid replacement therapy for opioid dependence. Cochrane Database Syst Rev(3): CD002209.

Mattick RP, Kimber J, et al. (2008). Buprenorphine maintenance versus placebo or methadone maintenance for opioid dependence. Cochrane Database Syst Rev(2): CD002207.

Max MB, Culnane M, et al. (1987). Amitriptyline relieves diabetic neuropathy pain in patients with normal or depressed mood. Neurology 37:589-596.

Mbaya P, Alam F, et al. (2007). Cardiovascular effects of high dose venlafaxine XL in patients with major depressive disorder. Human Psychopharmacology 22:129-133.

McCue RE, Waheed R, et al. (2006). Comparative effectiveness of second-generation antipsychotics and haloperidol in acute schizophrenia. British Journal of Psychiatry 189:433-440.

McEvoy JP, Stiller RL, et al. (1986). Plasma haloperidol levels drawn at neuroleptic threshold doses: a pilot study. Journal of Clinical Psychopharmacology 6:133-138.

McGough JJ and Barkley RA (2004). Diagnostic controversies in adult attention deficit hyperactivity disorder. Am J Psychiatry 161(11): 1948-1956.

McGrath PJ, Khan AY, et al. (2008). Response to a selective serotonin reuptake inhibitor (citalopram) in major depressive disorder with melancholic features: A STAR*D report. Journal of Clinical Psychiatry 69:1847-1855.

McGrath PJ, Stewart JW, et al. (2006). Tranylcypromine versus venlafaxine plus mirtazapine following three failed antidepressant medication trials for depression: a STAR*D report. American Journal of Psychiatry 163:1531-1541.

McIntyre RS, Cha DS, et al. (2012). A review of published evidence reporting on the efficacy and pharmacology of lurasidone." Expert Opin Pharmacother 13(11): 1653-1659.

McMahon FJ, Buervenich S, et al. (2006). Variation in the gene encoding the serotonin 2A receptor is associated with outcome of antidepressant treatment. American Journal of Human Genetics 78:804-814.

Meador KJ, Baker GA, et al. (2009). Cognitive function at 3 years of age after fetal exposure to antiepileptic drugs. N Engl J Med 360(16): 1597-1605.

Megarbane B, Hreiche R, et al. (2006). Does high-dose buprenorphine cause respiratory depression?: possible mechanisms and therapeutic consequences. Toxicological Reviews 25:79-85, 2006

Meltzer HY (2012). Clozapine: balancing safety with superior antipsychotic efficacy. Clin Schizophr Relat Psychoses 6(3): 134-144.

Meltzer HY, Alphs L, et. al. (2003). Clozapine treatment for suicidality in schizophrenia: International Suicide Prevention Trial (InterSePT). Archives of General Psychiatry 60:82-91.

Mentzel CL, Tenback DE, et al. (2012). Efficacy and safety of deep brain stimulation in patients with medication-induced tardive dyskinesia and/or dystonia: a systematic review. J Clin Psychiatry 73(11): 1434-1438.

Meszaros A, Czobor P, et al. (2007). Pharmacotherapy of adult Attention Deficit/Hyperactivity Disorder (ADHD): a systematic review. Psychiatria Hungarica 22:259-270.

Mets MA, van Deventer KR, et al. (2010). Critical appraisal of ramelteon in the treatment of insomnia. Nat Sci Sleep 2: 257-266.

Meyer JM, Simpson GM (1997). From chlorpromazine to olanzapine: a brief history of antipsychotics. Psychiatric Services 48:1137-1139.

MHRA (2006). Medicines and Healthcare products Regulatory Agency & Commission on Human Medicines. Risk of QT interval prolongation with methadone. Report No.: 31.

Miceli JJ, Glue P, et al. (2007). The effect of food on the absorption of oral ziprasidone. Psychopharmacology Bulletin 40:58-68.

Michelson D, Adler L, et al. (2003). Atomoxetine in adults with ADHD: two randomized, placebo-controlled studies. Biological Psychiatry 53:112-120.

Miklowitz DJ (2008). Adjunctive psychotherapy for bipolar disorder: state of the evidence. American Journal of Psychiatry 165:1408-1419.

Miklowitz DJ, Otto MW, et al. (2007). Psychosocial treatments for bipolar depression: a 1-year randomized trial from the Systematic Treatment Enhancement Program. Archives of General Psychiatry 64:419-426.

Miller LJ (2008). Prazosin for the treatment of posttraumatic stress disorder sleep disturbances. Pharmacotherapy 28:656-666.

Mills EJ, Wu P, et al. (2012). Comparisons of high-dose and combination nicotine replacement therapy, varenicline, and bupropion for smoking cessation: a systematic review and multiple treatment meta-analysis. Ann Med 44(6): 588-597.

Mitchell JM, Grossman LE, et al. (2012). The anticonvulsant levetiracetam potentiates alcohol consumption in non-treatment seeking alcohol abusers. J Clin Psychopharmacol 32(2): 269-272.

Mohammad OM, Osser DN (2014). The Psychopharmacology Algorithm Project at the Harvard South Shore Program: an algorithm for acute mania. Harv Rev Psychiatry 22(5): 274-94.

Mongia M and Hechtman L (2012). Cognitive behavior therapy for adults with attention-deficit/hyperactivity disorder: a review of recent randomized controlled trials. Curr Psychiatry Rep 14(5): 561-567.

Montejo AL, Llorca G, et al. (2001). Incidence of sexual dysfunction associated with antidepressant agents: a prospective multicenter study of 1022 outpatients. Spanish Working Group for the Study of Psychotropic-Related Sexual Dysfunction. Journal of Clinical Psychiatry 62(Suppl 3):10-21.

Moore GJ, Cortese BM, et al. (2009). A longitudinal study of the effects of lithium treatment on prefrontal and subgenual prefrontal gray matter volume in treatment-responsive bipolar disorder patients. J Clin Psychiatry 70(5): 699-705.

Moore TJ, Furberg CD, et al. (2011). Suicidal behavior and depression in smoking cessation treatments. PLoS One 6(11): e27016.

Morgenthaler TI, Silber MH (2002). Amnestic sleep-related eating disorder associated with zolpidem. Sleep Med 3(4): 323-327.

Mork A, Montezinho LP, et al. (2013). Vortioxetine (Lu AA21004), a novel multimodal antidepressant, enhances memory in rats. Pharmacol Biochem Behav 105: 41-50.

Morley KC, Teesson M, et al. (2006). Naltrexone versus acamprosate in the treatment of alcohol dependence: A multi-centre, randomized, double-blind, placebo-controlled trial. Addiction 101:1451-1462.

Morrato EH, Libby AM, et al. (2008). Frequency of provider contact after FDA advisory on risk of pediatric suicidality with SSRIs. American Journal of Psychiatry 165:42-50.

Movig KL, Leufkens HG, et al. (2002). Association between antidepressant drug use and hyponatraemia: a case-control study. Br J Clin Pharmacol 53(4): 363-369.

Mueller TI, Stout RL, et al. (1997). A double-blind, placebo-controlled pilot study of carbamazepine for the treatment of alcohol dependence. Alcohol Clin Exp Res 21(1): 86-92.

Mugunthan K, McGuire T, et al. (2011). Minimal interventions to decrease long-term use of benzodiazepines in primary care: a systematic review and meta-analysis. Br J Gen Pract 61(590): e573-578.

Murphy GM, Jr., Hollander SB, et al. (2004). Effects of the serotonin transporter gene promoter polymorphism on mirtazapine and paroxetine efficacy and adverse events in geriatric major depression. Archives of General Psychiatry 61:1163-1169.

Muzyk AJ, Rivelli SK, et al. (2012). Defining the role of baclofen for the treatment of alcohol dependence: a systematic review of the evidence. CNS Drugs 26(1): 69-78.

Nelson JC, Thase ME, et al. (2012). Efficacy of adjunctive aripiprazole in patients with major depressive disorder who showed minimal response to initial antidepressant therapy. Int Clin Psychopharmacol 27(3): 125-133.

Nestler EJ, Hyman SE, Malenka RC (2009). Molecular Neuropharmacology: A Foundation for Clinical Neuroscience, Second Edition. New York: McGraw-Hill Companies, Inc.

Nielsen J, Graff C, et al. (2011). Assessing QT interval prolongation and its associated risks with antipsychotics. CNS Drugs 25(6): 473-490.

Nierenberg AA, Fava M, et al. (2006). A comparison of lithium and T(3) augmentation following two failed medication treatments for depression: a STAR*D report. American Journal of Psychiatry 163:1519-1530.

Nunes PV, Forlenza OV, et al. (2007). Lithium and risk for Alzheimer's disease in elderly patients with bipolar disorder. British Journal of Psychiatry 190:359-360.

Nussbaum AM, Stroup TS (2012). Paliperidone palmitate for schizophrenia. Cochrane Database Syst Rev 6: CD008296.

Nutt DJ, Malizia AL (2001). New insights into the role of the GABA(A)-benzodiazepine receptor in psychiatric disorder. British Journal of Psychiatry 179:390-396.

Nyberg S, Eriksson B, et al. (1999). Suggested minimal effective dose of risperidone based on PET-measured D2 and 5-HT2A receptor occupancy in schizophrenic patients. American Journal of Psychiatry 156:869-875.

O'Donovan C, Garnham JS, et al. (2008). Antidepressant monotherapy in pre-bipolar depression; predictive value and inherent risk. Journal of Affective Disorders 107:293-298.

O'Donovan C, Kusumakar V, et al. (2002). Menstrual abnormalities and polycystic ovary syndrome in women taking valproate for bipolar mood disorder. Journal of Clinical Psychiatry 63:322-330.

O'Malley SS, Garbutt JC, et al. (2007). Efficacy of extended-release naltrexone in alcohol-dependent patients who are abstinent before treatment. Journal of Clinical Psychopharmacology 27:507-512.

Olfson M, Blanco C, et al. (2013). Trends in office-based treatment of adults with stimulants in the United States. J Clin Psychiatry 74(1): 43-50.

Olfson M, Marcus SC, et al. (2007). Treatment of schizophrenia with long-acting fluphenazine, haloperidol, or risperidone. Schizophrenia Bulletin 33:1379-1387.

Olmsted CL, Kockler DR (2008). Topiramate for alcohol dependence. Ann Pharmacother 42(10): 1475-1480.

Onghena P, Van Houdenhove B (1992). Antidepressant-induced analgesia in chronic non-malignant pain: a meta-analysis of 39 placebo-controlled studies. Pain 49:205-219.

Orriols L, Philip P, et al. (2011). Benzodiazepine-like hypnotics and the associated risk of road traffic accidents. Clin Pharmacol Ther 89(4): 595-601.

Ortenzi A, Paggi A, et al. (2008). Oxcarbazepine and adverse events: impact of age, dosage, metabolite serum concentrations and concomitant antiepileptic therapy. Functional Neurology 23:97-100.

Osser DN (2008). Cleaning up evidence-based psychopharmacology. Psychopharm Review 43:19-25.

Osser DN, Dunlop LR (2010). The Psychopharmacology Algorithm Project at the Harvard South Shore Program: an update on generalized social anxiety disorder. Psychopharm Review 45: 91-98.

Osser DN, Najarian DM, Dufresne RL (1999). Olanzapine increases weight and serum triglyceride levels. Journal of Clinical Psychiatry 60:767-770.

Osser DN, Renner JA, Bayog R (1999). Algorithms for the pharmacotherapy of anxiety disorders in patients with chemical abuse and dependence. Psychiatric Annals 29(5): 285-301.

Osser DN, Roudsari MJ, et al. (2013). The Psychopharmacology Algorithm Project at the Harvard South Shore Program: an update on schizophrenia. Harv Rev Psychiatry 21(1): 18-40.

Osser DN, Sigadel R (2001). Short-term inpatient pharmacotherapy of schizophrenia. Harv Rev Psychiatry 9(3): 89-104.

Oulis P, Konstantakopoulos G (2012). Efficacy and safety of pregabalin in the treatment of alcohol and benzodiazepine dependence. Expert Opin Investig Drugs 21(7): 1019-1029.

Pacchiarotti I, Bond DJ, et al. (2103). The International Society for Bipolar Disorders (ISBD) task force report on antidepressant use in bipolar disorders. Am J Psychiatry 170(11): 1249-62.

Palumbo DR, Sallee FR, et al. (2008). Clonidine for attention-deficit/hyperactivity disorder: I. Efficacy and tolerability outcomes. J Am Acad Child Adolesc Psychiatry 47(2): 180-188.

Pande AC, Crockatt JG, et al. (2000). Gabapentin in bipolar disorder: a placebo-controlled trial of adjunctive therapy. Gabapentin Bipolar Disorder Study Group. Bipolar Disorders 2:249-255.

Parr JM, Kavanagh DJ, et al. (2009). Effectiveness of current treatment approaches for benzodiazepine discontinuation: a meta-analysis. Addiction 104(1): 13-24.

PDR-Physicians' Desk Reference (2014). http://www.pdr.net.

Perlis RH, Welge JA, et al. (2006). Atypical antipsychotics in the treatment of mania: a meta-analysis of randomized, placebo-controlled trials. J Clin Psychiatry 67(4): 509-516.

Perry PJ, Zeilmann C, et al. (1994). Tricyclic antidepressant concentrations in plasma: an estimate of their sensitivity and specificity as a predictor of response. Journal of Clinical Psychopharmacology 14:230-240.

Perucca E (2006). Clinically relevant drug interactions with antiepileptic drugs. British Journal of Clinical Pharmacology 61:246-255.

Petrov I, Krogh J, et al. (2011). Meta-analysis of pharmacological therapy with acamprosate, naltrexone, and disulfiram--a systematic review. Ugeskr Laeger 173(48): 3103-3109.

Pettinati HM, O'Brien CP, et al. (2006). The status of naltrexone in the treatment of alcohol dependence: specific effects on heavy drinking. Journal of Clinical Psychopharmacology 26:610-625.

Pettinati HM, Oslin DW, et al. (2010). A double-blind, placebo-controlled trial combining sertraline and naltrexone for treating co-occurring depression and alcohol dependence. Am J Psychiatry 167(6): 668-675.

Pettinati HM, Silverman BL, et al. (2011). Efficacy of extended-release naltrexone in patients with relatively higher severity of alcohol dependence. Alcohol Clin Exp Res 35(10): 1804-1811.

Pettinati HM, Volpicelli JR, et al. (2000). Sertraline treatment for alcohol dependence: interactive effects of medication and alcoholic subtype. Alcohol Clin Exp Res 24(7): 1041-1049.

Phansalkar S, Osser DN (2009). Optimizing Clozapine Treatment: Part I. Psychopharm Review 44:1-8.

Phansalkar S, Osser DN (2009). Optimizing Clozapine Treatment: Part II. Psychopharm Review 44:9-15.

Phelps J (2008). The bipolar spectrum, in Parker G (ed.), Bipolar II Disorder. Modeling, Measuring, and Managing. Cambridge, UK: Cambridge University Press.

Pigott TA, Carson WH, et al. (2003). Aripiprazole for the prevention of relapse in stabilized patients with chronic schizophrenia: a placebo-controlled 26-week study. Journal of Clinical Psychiatry 64:1048-1056.

Piper ME, Smith SS, et al. (2009). A randomized placebo-controlled clinical trial of 5 smoking cessation pharmacotherapies. Arch Gen Psychiatry 66(11): 1253-1262.

Popper CW (1997). Antidepressants in the treatment of attention-deficit/hyperactivity disorder. Journal of Clinical Psychiatry 58(Suppl 14):14-29.

Porcelli S, Fabbri C, et al. (2012). Meta-analysis of serotonin transporter gene promoter polymorphism (5-HTTLPR) association with antidepressant efficacy. Eur Neuropsychopharmacol 22(4): 239-258.

Post RM (1990). Sensitization and kindling perspectives for the course of affective illness: toward a new treatment with the anticonvulsant carbamazepine. Pharmacopsychiatry 23(1): 3-17.

Post RM, Altshuler LL, et al. (2006). Mood switch in bipolar depression: comparison of adjunctive venlafaxine, bupropion and sertraline. British Journal of Psychiatry 189:124-131.

Post RM, Uhde TW, et al. (1982). Kindling and carbamazepine in affective illness. J Nerv Ment Dis 170(12): 717-731.

Potkin SG (2011). Asenapine: a clinical overview. J Clin Psychiatry 72 Suppl 1: 14-18.

Praharaj SK, Jana AK, et al. (2011). Metformin for olanzapine-induced weight gain: a systematic review and meta-analysis. Br J Clin Pharmacol 71(3): 377-382.

Pratoomsri W, Yatham LN, et al. (2006). Oxcarbazepine in the treatment of bipolar disorder: a review. Canadian Journal of Psychiatry 51:540-545.

Prince JB, Wilens TE, et al. (2000). A controlled study of nortriptyline in children and adolescents with attention deficit hyperactivity disorder. Journal of Child and Adolescent Psychopharmacology 10:193-204.

Prochaska JJ, Hilton JF (2012). Risk of cardiovascular serious adverse events associated with varenicline use for tobacco cessation: systematic review and meta-analysis. BMJ 344: e2856.

Quiroz JA, Yatham LN, et al. (2010). Risperidone long-acting injectable monotherapy in the maintenance treatment of bipolar I disorder. Biol Psychiatry 68(2): 156-162.

Quitkin FM, Stewart JW, et al. (1993). Columbia atypical depression. A subgroup of depressives with better response to MAOI than to tricyclic antidepressants or placebo. British Journal of Psychiatry. (Suppl 21): 30-34.

Raja M (2007). Improvement or worsening of psychotic symptoms after treatment with low doses of aripiprazole. International Journal of Neuropsychopharmacology 10:107-110.

Raskin J, Goldstein DJ, et al. (2003). Duloxetine in the long-term treatment of major depressive disorder. Journal of Clinical Psychiatry 64:1237-1244.

Raskind MA, Peskind ER, et al. (2007). A parallel group placebo controlled study of prazosin for trauma nightmares and sleep disturbance in combat veterans with post-traumatic stress disorder. Biological Psychiatry 61:928-934.

Raskind MA, Peterson K, et al. (2013). A Trial of Prazosin for Combat Trauma PTSD With Nightmares in Active-Duty Soldiers Returned From Iraq and Afghanistan. Am J Psychiatry.

Ray WA, Chung CP, et al. (2009). Atypical antipsychotic drugs and the risk of sudden cardiac death. New England Journal of Medicine 360:225-235.

Ray WA, Meredith S, et al. (2004). Cyclic antidepressants and the risk of sudden cardiac death. Clinical Pharmacology and Therapeutics 75:234-241.

Reddy S, Kane C, et al. (2010). Clinical utility of desvenlafaxine 50 mg/d for treating MDD: a review of two randomized placebo-controlled trials for the practicing physician. Curr Med Res Opin 26(1): 139-150.

Reynolds CF, Frank E, et al. (1999). Nortriptyline and interpersonal psychotherapy as maintenance therapies for recurrent major depression: a randomized controlled trial in patients older than 59 years. Journal of the American Medical Association 281:39-45.

Richelson E (2003). Interactions of antidepressants with neurotransmitter transporters and receptors and their clinical relevance. Journal of Clinical Psychiatry 64(Suppl 13):5-12.

Rickels K, Athanasiou M, et al. (2009). Evidence for efficacy and tolerability of vilazodone in the treatment of major depressive disorder: a randomized, double-blind, placebo-controlled trial. J Clin Psychiatry 70(3): 326-333.

Rihmer Z, Dome P, et al. (2013). Antidepressant response and subthreshold bipolarity in "unipolar" major depressive disorder: implications for practice and drug research. J Clin Psychopharmacol 33(4): 449-452.

Risbood V, Lee JR, et al. (2012). Lurasidone: an atypical antipsychotic for schizophrenia. Ann Pharmacother 46(7-8): 1033-1046.

Rochon PA, Normand SL, et al. (2008). Antipsychotic therapy and short-term serious events in older adults with dementia. Archives of Internal Medicine 168:1090-1096.

Rosenbaum JF, Arana GW, et al. (2005). Handbook of Psychiatric Drug Therapy, Fifth Edition. Philadelphia, PA: Lippincott Williams & Wilkins.

Rosner S, Hackl-Herrwerth A, et al. (2010). Acamprosate for alcohol dependence." Cochrane Database Syst Rev(9): CD004332.

Ross RG (2006). Psychotic and manic-like symptoms during stimulant treatment of attention deficit hyperactivity disorder. Am J Psychiatry 163(7): 1149-1152.

Roth T, Seiden D, et al. (2006). Effects of Ramelteon on patient-reported sleep latency in older adults with chronic insomnia. Sleep Medicine 7:312-318.

Rubio G, Jimenez-Arriero MA, et al. (2001). Naltrexone versus acamprosate: one year follow-up of alcohol dependence treatment. Alcohol and Alcoholism 36:419-425.

Rubio G, Martinez-Gras I, et al. (2009). Modulation of impulsivity by topiramate: implications for the treatment of alcohol dependence. J Clin Psychopharmacol 29(6): 584-589.

Rush AJ, Trivedi MH, et al. (2006). Acute and longer-term outcomes in depressed outpatients requiring one or several treatment steps: a STAR*D report. American Journal of Psychiatry 163:1905-1917.

Rush AJ, Trivedi MH, et al. (2011). Combining medications to enhance depression outcomes (CO-MED): acute and long-term outcomes of a single-blind randomized study. Am J Psychiatry 168(7): 689-701.

Saarto T, Wiffen PJ (2007). Antidepressants for neuropathic pain. Cochrane Database of Systematic Reviews CD005454.

Sachs GS (1990). Use of clonazepam for bipolar affective disorder. J Clin Psychiatry 51 Suppl: 31-34; discussion 50-33.

Sachs GS, Nierenberg AA, et al. (2007). Effectiveness of adjunctive antidepressant treatment for bipolar depression. New England Journal of Medicine 356:1711-1722.

Sachs GS, Rosenbaum JF, et al. (1990). Adjunctive clonazepam for maintenance treatment of bipolar affective disorder. J Clin Psychopharmacol 10(1): 42-47.

Sallee FR and Eaton K (2010). Guanfacine extended-release for attention-deficit/hyperactivity disorder (ADHD). Expert Opin Pharmacother 11(15): 2549-2556.

Salzman C, Glick I, et al. (2010). The 7 sins of psychopharmacology. J Clin Psychopharmacol 30(6): 653-655.

Sanger DJ (2004). The pharmacology and mechanisms of action of new generation, non-benzodiazepine hypnotic agents. CNS Drugs 18(Suppl 1):9-15.

Sarris J, Mischoulon D, et al. (2012). Omega-3 for bipolar disorder: meta-analyses of use in mania and bipolar depression. J Clin Psychiatry 73(1): 81-86.

Sass H, Soyka M, et al. (1996). Relapse prevention by acamprosate. Results from a placebo-controlled study on alcohol dependence. Archives of General Psychiatry 53:673-680.

Sateia MJ, Kirby-Long P, et al. (2008). Efficacy and clinical safety of Ramelteon: an evidence-based review. Sleep Medicine Reviews 12:319-332.

Satel SL, Nelson JC (1989). Stimulants in the treatment of depression: a critical overview. Journal of Clinical Psychiatry 50:241-249.

Satterthwaite TD, Wolf DH, et al. (2008). A meta-analysis of the risk of acute extrapyramidal symptoms with intramuscular antipsychotics for the treatment of agitation. Journal of Clinical Psychiatry 69:1869-1879.

Schneeweiss S, Setoguchi S, et al. (2007). Risk of death associated with the use of conventional versus atypical antipsychotic drugs among elderly patients. Canadian Medical Association Journal 176:627-632.

Schneider LS, Dagerman KS, et al. (2005): Risk of death with atypical antipsychotic drug treatment for dementia: meta-analysis of randomized placebo-controlled trials. Journal of the American Medical Association 294:1934-1943

Schneider LS, Tariot PN, et al. (2006). Effectiveness of atypical antipsychotic drugs in patients with Alzheimer's disease. New England Journal of Medicine 355:1525-1538.

Schueler YB, Koesters M, et al. (2011). A systematic review of duloxetine and venlafaxine in major depression, including unpublished data. Acta Psychiatr Scand 123(4): 247-265.

Schutte-Rodin S, Broch L, et al. (2008). Clinical guideline for the evaluation and management of chronic insomnia in adults. J Clin Sleep Med 4(5): 487-504.

Schwieler L, Linderholm KR, et al. (2008). Clozapine interacts with the glycine site of the NMDA receptor: electrophysiological studies of dopamine neurons in the rat ventral tegmental area. Life Sci 83(5-6): 170-175.

Seeman P (1992). Dopamine receptor sequences. Therapeutic levels of neuroleptics occupy D2 receptors, clozapine occupies D4. Neuropsychopharmacology 7(4): 261-284.

Seeman P (2002). Atypical antipsychotics: mechanism of action. Can J Psychiatry 47(1): 27-38.

Serretti A, Drago A, et al. (2009). Lithium pharmacodynamics and pharmacogenetics: focus on inositol mono phosphatase (IMPase), inositol poliphosphatase (IPPase) and glycogen sinthase kinase 3 beta (GSK-3 beta). Curr Med Chem 16(15): 1917-1948.

Serretti A, Mandelli L (2010). Antidepressants and body weight: a comprehensive review and meta-analysis. J Clin Psychiatry 71(10): 1259-1272.

Sethi PK, Khandelwal DC (2005). Zolpidem at supratherapeutic doses can cause drug abuse, dependence and withdrawal seizure. Journal of the Association of the Physicians of India 53:139-140.

Severus WE, Kleindienst N, et al. (2008). What is the optimal serum lithium level in the long-term treatment of bipolar disorder--a review? Bipolar Disorders 10:231-237.

Shah RR (2005). Drug-induced QT dispersion: does it predict the risk of torsade de pointes? Journal of Electrocardiology 38:10-18.

Shaldubina A, Agam G, et al. (2001). The mechanism of lithium action: state of the art, ten years later. Progress in Neuropsychopharmacology and Biological Psychiatry 25:855-866.

Shamir E, Barak Y, et al. (2001). Melatonin treatment of tardive dyskinesia: a double-blind, placebo-controlled, crossover study. Arch Gen Psychiatry 58(11): 1049-52.

Shaw M, Hodgkins P, et al. (2012). A systematic review and analysis of long-term outcomes in attention deficit hyperactivity disorder: effects of treatment and non-treatment. BMC Med 10: 99.

Sheehan DV, Croft HA, et al. (2009). Extended-release Trazodone in Major Depressive Disorder: A Randomized, Double-blind, Placebo-controlled Study. Psychiatry (Edgmont) 6(5): 20-33.

Shevell M (1997). Pemoline associated hepatic failure: a critical analysis of the literature. Pediatr Neurol 16(4): 353.

Sicard MN, Zai CC, et al. (2010). Polymorphisms of the HTR2C gene and antipsychotic-induced weight gain: an update and meta-analysis. Pharmacogenomics 11(11): 1561-1571.

Sikich L, Frazier JA, et al. (2008). Double-blind comparison of first- and second-generation antipsychotics in early-onset schizophrenia and schizo-affective disorder: findings from the treatment of early-onset schizophrenia spectrum disorders (TEOSS) study. American Journal of Psychiatry 165:1420-1431.

Silagy C, Lancaster T, et al. (2004). Nicotine replacement therapy for smoking cessation. Cochrane Database of Systematic Reviews CD000146.

Silagy C, Mant D, et al. (2000). Nicotine replacement therapy for smoking cessation. Cochrane Database of Systematic Reviews CD000146.

Simpson TL, Saxon AJ, et al. (2009). A pilot trial of the alpha-1 adrenergic antagonist, prazosin, for alcohol dependence. Alcohol Clin Exp Res 33(2): 255-263.

Singh S, Loke YK, et al. (2011). Risk of serious adverse cardiovascular events associated with varenicline: a systematic review and meta-analysis. CMAJ 183(12): 1359-1366.

Siriwardena AN, Qureshi Z, et al. (2006). GPs' attitudes to benzodiazepines and 'Z-drug' prescribing: a barrier to implementation of evidence and guidance on hypnotics. British Journal of General Practice 56:964-967.

Sivertsen B, Omvik S, et al. (2006). Cognitive behavioral therapy vs. zopiclone for treatment of chronic primary insomnia in older adults: a randomized controlled trial. Journal of the American Medical Association 295:2851-2858.

Smink BE, Egberts AC, et al. (2010). The relationship between benzodiazepine use and traffic accidents: A systematic literature review. CNS Drugs 24(8): 639-653.

Soares-Weiser K, Fernandez HH (2007). Tardive dyskinesia. Seminars in Neurology 27:159-169.

Soares-Weiser K, Maayan N, et al. (2011). Vitamin E for neuroleptic-induced tardive dyskinesia. Cochrane Database Syst Rev(2): CD000209.

Sommer IE, de Witte L, et al. (2012). Nonsteroidal anti-inflammatory drugs in schizophrenia: ready for practice or a good start? A meta-analysis. J Clin Psychiatry 73(4): 414-419.

Sommer IE, van Westrhenen R, et al. (2014). Efficacy of anti-inflammatory agents to improve symptoms in patients with schizophrenia: an update. Schizophr Bull 40(1): 181-191.

Soyka M (2012). Buprenorphine and buprenorphine/naloxone soluble-film for treatment of opioid dependence. Expert Opin Drug Deliv 9(11): 1409-1417.

Spencer T, Biederman J, et al. (2005). A large, double-blind, randomized clinical trial of methylphenidate in the treatment of adults with attention-deficit/hyperactivity disorder. Biol Psychiatry 57(5): 456-63.

Spielmans GI (2008). Duloxetine does not relieve painful physical symptoms in depression: a meta-analysis. Psychother Psychosom 77(1): 12-16.

Spielmans GI, Berman MI, et al. (2013). Adjunctive atypical antipsychotic treatment for major depressive disorder: a meta-analysis of depression, quality of life, and safety outcomes. PLoS Med 10(3): e1001403.

Spina E, Scordo MG, et al. (2003). Metabolic drug interactions with new psychotropic agents. Fundamental and Clinical Pharmacology 17:517-538.

Srisurapanont M, Jarusuraisin N (2005). Opioid antagonists for alcohol dependence. Cochrane Database of Systematic Reviews CD001867.

Stagnitti MN (2008). Antidepressants prescribed by medical doctors in office based and outpatient settings by specialty for the U.S. civilian non-institutionalized population, 2002 and 2005. Statistical Brief #206. Medical Expenditure Panel Survey. Agency for Healthcare Research and Quality.

Stahl SM (2000). The 7 habits of highly effective psychopharmacologists: overview. J Clin Psychiatry 61(4): 242-243.

Stahl SM (2001). "Hit-and-run" actions at dopamine receptors, part 1: Mechanism of action of atypical antipsychotics. J Clin Psychiatry 62(9): 670-671.

Stahl SM (2008). Stahl's Essential Psychopharmacology: Neuroscientific Basis and Practical Applications. 3rd Edition. New York, NY: Cambridge University Press.

Stahl SM, Grady MM (2003). Differences in mechanism of action between current and future antidepressants. Journal of Clinical Psychiatry 64(Suppl 13):13-17.

Stamm TJ, Lewitzka U, et al. (2014). Supraphysiological doses of levothyroxine as adjunctive therapy in bipolar depression: a randomized, double-blind, placebo-controlled study. J Clin Psychiatry 75(2): 162-68.

Stead LF, Perera R, et al. (2012). Nicotine replacement therapy for smoking cessation. Cochrane Database Syst Rev 11: CD000146.

Sterke CS, Ziere G, et al. (2012). Dose-response relationship between Selective Serotonin Reuptake Inhibitors and Injurious Falls: A study in Nursing Home Residents with Dementia. Br J Clin Pharmacol 73(5):812-20.

Stoner SC, Pace HA (2012). Asenapine: a clinical review of a second-generation antipsychotic. Clin Ther 34(5): 1023-1040.

Straus SM, Bleumink GS, et al. (2004). Antipsychotics and the risk of sudden cardiac death. Archives of Internal Medicine 164:1293-1297.

Suh JJ, Pettinati HM, et al. (2006). The status of disulfiram: a half of a century later. Journal of Clinical Psychopharmacology 26:290-302.

Sultzer DL, Davis SM, et al. (2008). Clinical symptom responses to atypical antipsychotic medications in Alzheimer's disease: phase 1 outcomes from the CATIE-AD effectiveness trial. American Journal of Psychiatry 165:844-854.

Summerfelt WT, Meltzer HY (1998). Efficacy vs. effectiveness in psychiatric research. Psychiatric Services 49:834-835.

Sun H, Kennedy WP, et al. (2013). Effects of suvorexant, an orexin receptor agonist, on sleep parameters as measured by polysomnography in healthy men. Sleep 36(2): 259-67.

Sung SC, Haley CL, et al. (2012). The impact of chronic depression on acute and long-term outcomes in a randomized trial comparing selective serotonin reuptake inhibitor monotherapy versus each of 2 different antidepressant medication combinations. J Clin Psychiatry 73(7): 967-976.

Suppes T, Vieta E, et al. (2009). Maintenance treatment for patients with bipolar I disorder: results from a north american study of quetiapine in combination with lithium or divalproex (trial 127). Am J Psychiatry 166(4): 476-488.

Suzuki T, Uchida H, et al. (2007). How effective is it to sequentially switch among olanzapine, quetiapine and risperidone?--A randomized, open-label study of algorithm-based antipsychotic treatment to patients with symptomatic schizophrenia in the real-world clinical setting. Psychopharmacology 195:285-295.

Suzuki Y, Fukui N, et al. (2012). QT prolongation of the antipsychotic risperidone is predominantly related to its 9-hydroxy metabolite paliperidone. Hum Psychopharmacol 27(1): 39-42.

Svanstrom H, Pasternak B, et al. (2012). Use of varenicline for smoking cessation and risk of serious cardiovascular events: nationwide cohort study. BMJ 345: e7176.

Swann AC, Lafer B, et al. (2013). Bipolar mixed states: an international society for bipolar disorders task force report of symptom structure, course of illness, and diagnosis. Am J Psychiatry 170(1): 31-42.

Swartz MS, Stroup TS, et al. (2008). What CATIE found: results from the schizophrenia trial. Psychiatr Serv 59(5): 500-506.

Tahir TA, Eeles E, et al. (2010). A randomized controlled trial of quetiapine versus placebo in the treatment of delirium. J Psychosom Res 69(5): 485-490.

Takahata K, Ito H, et al. (2012). Striatal and extrastriatal dopamine D(2) receptor occupancy by the partial agonist antipsychotic drug aripiprazole in the human brain: a positron emission tomography study with [(1)(1)C]raclopride and [(1)(1)C]FLB457. Psychopharmacology (Berl) 222(1): 165-172.

Tang M, Osser DN (2012). The Psychopharmacology Algorithm Project at the Harvard South Shore Program: 2012 update on psychotic depression. Journal of Mood Disorders 2(4): 168-179.

Tang SW, Helmeste D, et al. (2012). Is neurogenesis relevant in depression and in the mechanism of antidepressant drug action? A critical review. World J Biol Psychiatry 13(6): 402-412.

Tarazi FI, Stahl SM (2012). Iloperidone, asenapine and lurasidone: a primer on their current status." Expert Opin Pharmacother 13(13): 1911-1922.

Tarr GP, Glue P, et al. (2011). Comparative efficacy and acceptability of mood stabilizer and second generation antipsychotic monotherapy for acute mania--a systematic review and meta-analysis. J Affect Disord 134(1-3): 14-19.

Tarsy D, Lungu C, et al. (2011). Epidemiology of tardive dyskinesia before and during the era of modern antipsychotic drugs. Handb Clin Neurol 100: 601-616.

Taylor FB, Lowe K, et al. (2006). Daytime prazosin reduces psychological distress to trauma specific cues in civilian trauma posttraumatic stress disorder. Biological Psychiatry 59:577-581.

Taylor FB, Martin P, et al. (2008). Prazosin effects on objective sleep measures and clinical symptoms in civilian trauma posttraumatic stress disorder: a placebo-controlled study. Biological Psychiatry 63:629-632.

Taylor MJ, Freemantle N, et al. (2006). Early onset of selective serotonin reuptake inhibitor antidepressant action: systematic review and meta-analysis. Arch Gen Psychiatry 63(11): 1217-1223.

Thase ME (2012). The role of monoamine oxidase inhibitors in depression treatment guidelines. J Clin Psychiatry 73 Suppl 1: 10-16.

Thase ME, Jonas A, et al. (2008). Aripiprazole monotherapy in nonpsychotic bipolar I depression: results of 2 randomized, placebo-controlled studies. J Clin Psychopharmacol 28(1): 13-20.

Thase ME, Macfadden W, et al. (2006). Efficacy of quetiapine monotherapy in bipolar I and II depression: a double-blind, placebo-controlled study (the BOLDER II study). Journal of Clinical Psychopharmacology 26:600-609.

Tohen M, Calabrese JR, et al. (2006). Randomized, placebo-controlled trial of olanzapine as maintenance therapy in patients with bipolar I disorder responding to acute treatment with olanzapine. Am J Psychiatry 163(2): 247-256.

Tohen M, Chengappa KN, et al. (2004). Relapse prevention in bipolar I disorder: 18-month comparison of olanzapine plus mood stabiliser v. mood stabiliser alone. Br J Psychiatry 184: 337-345.

Tohen M, Vieta E (2009). Antipsychotic agents in the treatment of bipolar mania. Bipolar Disord 11 Suppl 2: 45-54.

Tohen M, Vieta E, et al. (2003). Efficacy of olanzapine and olanzapine-fluoxetine combination in the treatment of bipolar I depression. Arch Gen Psychiatry 60(11): 1079-1088.

Tohen M, Zarate CA Jr. (1998). Antipsychotic agents and bipolar disorder. J Clin Psychiatry 59 Suppl 1: 38-48; discussion 49.

Tonstad S, Tonnesen P, et al. (2006). Effect of maintenance therapy with varenicline on smoking cessation: a randomized controlled trial. Journal of the American Medical Association 296:64-71.

Trivedi M, Thase ME, et al. (2008). Adjunctive aripiprazole in major depressive disorder: analysis of efficacy and safety in patients with anxious and atypical features. Journal of Clinical Psychiatry 69:1928-1936.

Trivedi MH, Fava M, et al. (2006). Medication augmentation after the failure of SSRIs for depression. New England Journal of Medicine 354:1243-1252.

Trivedi MH, Rush AJ, et al. (2001). Do bupropion SR and sertraline differ in their effects on anxiety in depressed patients? J Clin Psychiatry 62(10): 776-781.

Trollor JN, Chen X, et al. (2009). Neuroleptic malignant syndrome associated with atypical antipsychotic drugs. CNS Drugs 23(6): 477-492.

Tsai JH, Yang P, et al. (2009). Zolpidem-induced amnesia and somnambulism: rare occurrences? Eur Neuropsychopharmacol 19(1): 74-76.

Turner EH, Matthews AM, et al. (2008). Selective publication of antidepressant trials and its influence on apparent efficacy. N Engl J Med 358(3): 252-260.

Turner EH, Rosenthal R (2008). Efficacy of antidepressants. BMJ 336(7643): 516-517.

Vajda FJ, Graham J, et al. (2012). Teratogenicity of the newer antiepileptic drugs--the Australian experience. J Clin Neurosci 19(1): 57-59.

van Harten PN, Tenback DE (2011). Tardive dyskinesia: clinical presentation and treatment. Int Rev Neurobiol 98: 187-210.

Van Winkel R, De Hert M, et al. (2006). Screening for diabetes and other metabolic abnormalities in patients with schizophrenia and schizoaffective disorder: evaluation of incidence and screening methods. Journal of Clinical Psychiatry 67:1493-1500.

Vasudev A, Macritchie K, et al. (2011). Oxcarbazepine for acute affective episodes in bipolar disorder. Cochrane Database Syst Rev(12): CD004857.

Verdel BM, Souverein PC, et al. (2010). Use of antidepressant drugs and risk of osteoporotic and non-osteoporotic fractures. Bone 47(3): 604-609.

REFERENCES

Victorri-Vigneau C, Dailly E, et al. (2007). Evidence of zolpidem abuse and dependence: results of the French Centre for Evaluation and Information on Pharmacodependence (CEIP) network survey. British Journal of Clinical Pharmacology 64:198-209.

Vieta E, Goikolea JM, et al. (2003). 1-year follow-up of patients treated with risperidone and topiramate for a manic episode. Journal of Clinical Psychiatry 64:834-839.

Vieta E, Manuel Goikolea, J, et al. (2006). A double-blind, randomized, placebo-controlled, prophylaxis study of adjunctive gabapentin for bipolar disorder. Journal of Clinical Psychiatry 67:473-477.

Vieta E, Sanchez-Moreno J, et al. (2003). Adjunctive topiramate in bipolar II disorder. World Journal of Biological Psychiatry 4:172-176.

Vieta E, Suppes T, et al. (2008). Efficacy and safety of quetiapine in combination with lithium or divalproex for maintenance of patients with bipolar I disorder (international trial 126). J Affect Disord 109(3): 251-263.

Viguera AC, Koukopoulos A, et al. (2007). Teratogenicity and anti-convulsants: lessons from neurology to psychiatry. Journal of Clinical Psychiatry 68(Suppl 9):29-33.

Voronin K, Randall P, et al. (2008). Aripiprazole effects on alcohol consumption and subjective reports in a clinical laboratory paradigm--possible influence of self-control. Alcohol Clin Exp Res 32(11): 1954-1961.

Waal HJ (1967). Propranolol-induced depression. British Medical Journal 2:50.

Wagner AK, Zhang F, et al. (2004). Benzodiazepine use and hip fractures in the elderly: who is at greatest risk? Archives of Internal Medicine 164:1567-1572.

Wagner KD, Redden L, et al. (2009). A double-blind, randomized, placebo-controlled trial of divalproex extended-release in the treatment of bipolar disorder in children and adolescents. J Am Acad Child Adolesc Psychiatry 48(5): 519-532.

Walsh BT, Seidman SN, et al. (2002). Placebo response in studies of major depression: variable, substantial, and growing. JAMA 287(14): 1840-1847.

Wang PS, Schneeweiss S, et al. (2005). Risk of death in elderly users of conventional vs. atypical antipsychotic medications. New England Journal of Medicine 353:2335-2341.

Wang SM, Han C, et al. (2012). Paliperidone: a review of clinical trial data and clinical implications." Clin Drug Investig 32(8): 497-512.

Washton AM, Gold MS, et al. (1984). Successful use of naltrexone in addicted physicians and business executives. Advances in Alcohol and Substance Abuse 4:89-96.

Weiden PJ (2012). Iloperidone for the treatment of schizophrenia: an updated clinical review." Clin Schizophr Relat Psychoses 6(1): 34-44.

Weisler RH, Kalali AH, et al. (2004). A multicenter, randomized, double-blind, placebo-controlled trial of extended-release carbamazepine capsules as monotherapy for bipolar disorder patients with manic or mixed episodes. Journal of Clinical Psychiatry 65:478-484.

Weisler RH, Keck PE, et al. (2005). Extended-release carbmazepine capsules as monotherapy for acute mania in bipolar disorder: a multicenter, randomized, double-blind, placebo-controlled trial. Journal of Clinical Psychiatry 66:323-330.

Whitworth AB, Fischer F, et al. (1996). Comparison of acamprosate and placebo in long-term treatment of alcohol dependence. Lancet 347:1438-1442.

REFERENCES

WHO-World Health Organization (2011). Essential Medicines World Health Organization Model List, 17th edition: http://apps.who.int/iris/bitstream/10665/70640/1/a95053_eng.pdf

Wilens TE (2004). Impact of ADHD and its treatment on substance abuse in adults. Journal of Clinical Psychiatry 65(Suppl 3):38-45.

Wilens TE, Biederman J, et al. (1996). Six-week, double-blind, placebo-controlled study of desipramine for adult attention deficit hyperactivity disorder. American Journal of Psychiatry 153:1147-1153.

Wilens TE, Bukstein O, et al. (2012). A controlled trial of extended-release guanfacine and psychostimulants for attention-deficit/hyperactivity disorder. J Am Acad Child Adolesc Psychiatry 51(1): 74-85 e72.

Wilens TE, Faraone SV, et al. (2003): Does stimulant therapy of attention-deficit/hyperactivity disorder beget later substance abuse? A meta-analytic review of the literature. Pediatrics 111:179-185.

Wilens TE, Spencer TJ, et al. (2001) A controlled clinical trial of bupropion for attention deficit hyperactivity disorder in adults. Am J Psychiatry. Feb;158(2):282-8.

Willcutt EG (2012). The prevalence of DSM-IV attention-deficit/hyperactivity disorder: a meta-analytic review. Neurotherapeutics 9(3): 490-499.

Williams SG, Alinejad NA, et al. (2010). Statistically significant increase in weight caused by low-dose quetiapine. Pharmacotherapy 30(10): 1011-1015.

Wingo AP and Ghaemi SN (2008). Frequency of stimulant treatment and of stimulant-associated mania/hypomania in bipolar disorder patients. Psychopharmacol Bull 41(4): 37-47.

Wisniewski SR, Fava M, et al. (2007). Acceptability of second-step treatments to depressed outpatients: a STAR*D report. American Journal of Psychiatry 164:753-760.

Wisniewski SR, Rush AJ, et al. (2009). Can phase III trial results of antidepressant medications be generalized to clinical practice? A STAR*D report. Am J Psychiatry 166(5): 599-607.

Wohlreich MM, Mallinckrodt CH, et al. (2007). Duloxetine for the treatment of major depressive disorder: safety and tolerability associated with dose escalation. Depression and Anxiety 24:41-52.

Wu RR, Zhao JP, et al. (2008). Lifestyle intervention and metformin for treatment of antipsychotic-induced weight gain: a randomized controlled trial. Journal of the American Medical Association 299:185-193.

Yildiz A, Gonul, AS, Tamam L (2002). Mechanism of Actions of Antidepressants: Beyond the Receptors. Bull Clin Psychopharmacology 12: 194-200.

Yoon SJ, Pae CU, et al. (2006). Mirtazapine for patients with alcohol dependence and comorbid depressive disorders: a multicentre, open label study. Prog Neuropsychopharmacol Biol Psychiatry 30(7): 1196-1201.

Young JL, Sarkis E, et al. (2011). Once-daily treatment with atomoxetine in adults with attention-deficit/hyperactivity disorder: a 24-week, randomized, double-blind, placebo-controlled trial. Clin Neuropharmacol 34(2): 51-60.

Yury CA, Fisher JE (2007). Meta-analysis of the effectiveness of atypical antipsychotics for the treatment of behavioral problems in persons with dementia. Psychotherapy and Psychosomatics 76:213-218.

Zacher JL, Roche-Desilets J (2005). Hypotension secondary to the combination of intramuscular olanzapine and intramuscular lorazepam. Journal of Clinical Psychiatry 66:1614-1615.

REFERENCES

Zarate CA Jr., Singh JB, et al. (2006). A randomized trial of an N-methyl-D-aspartate antagonist in treatment-resistant major depression. Arch Gen Psychiatry 63(8): 856-864.

Ziere G, Dieleman JP, et al. (2008). Selective serotonin reuptake inhibiting antidepressants are associated with an increased risk of nonvertebral fractures. J Clin Psychopharmacol 28(4): 411-417.

Zivin K, Pfeiffer PN, et al. (2013). Evaluation of the FDA warning against prescribing citalopram at doses exceeding 40 mg. Am J Psychiatry 170(6): 642-650.

INDEX

Made in the USA
Lexington, KY
01 July 2015